Essential MCQs on

Biostatistics and Epidemiology

(For MBBS, PGMEE and USMLE)

Essential MCQs on

Biostatistics and Epidemiology

(For MBBS, PGMEE and USMLE)

K.S. Negi
Associate Professor
Department of Community Medicine
Himalayan Institute of Medical Sciences
Swami Ram Nagar (Jolly Grant)
Dehradun (Uttaranchal)
INDIA

PEEPEE
PUBLISHERS AND DISTRIBUTORS (P) LTD.

Essential MCQs on Biostatistics and Epidemiology
(for MBBS, PGMEE and USMLE)

Published by
Pawaninder P. Vij and Anupam Vij
Peepee Publishers and Distributors (P) Ltd.
Head Office: 160, Shakti Vihar, Pitam Pura,
Delhi-110 034 (India)
Correspondence Address:
7/31, First Floor, Ansari Road, Daryaganj
New Delhi-110 002 (India)
Ph: 65195868, 23246245, 9811156083
e-mail: peepee160@yahoo.co.in
e-mail: peepee160@rediffmail.com
e-mail: peepee160@gmail.com
www.peepeepub.com

First Edition: 2006
Reprint: 2017

ISBN: 81-88867-66-7

Foreword

It gives me a great pleasure to write a foreword for a book entitled *"Essential MCQs on Biostatistics and Epidemiology"* diligently and intelligently compiled by Dr. K.S. Negi, Associate Professor, Department of Community Medicine, Himalayan Institute of Medical Sciences, Swami Ram Nagar, Dehradun (Uttaranchal).

Dr. Negi has put in a lot of effort and I am sure that the book will eminently serve the purpose and benefit to those seeking admissions to postgraduate medical degrees, as it is essential to sharpen their knowledge and success in the competitive examinations.

I wish all success to this endeavour.

Prof. U.C. Sharma
Principal
Himalayan Institute of Medical Sciences
and Dean, Faculty of Medicine
HNB Garhwal University
Srinagar (Garhwal)
Uttaranchal (India)

Preface

"One can help other(s) when able to help oneself"

Every medical graduate aspires to obtain postgraduate (MD/MS) degree. To fulfill this aspiration a systematic and thorough study is required. Besides the sound knowledge it is essential for students to prepare themselves for MCQs (Multiple Choice Questions) with full confidence and determination. As the MCQs are considered the most consistent, and reliable method to judge the student's knowledge, reasoning ability, skill and understanding of the basics of the subject.

This book has been prepared with a view to provide large volume of subject-matter particularly Biostatistics and Epidemiology. It consists of more than 700 questions arranged chapterwise. All types of questions, which have been asked in the recent past in PGMEE and USMLE, or are likely to be asked in entrance examination, have been included. The answers are given at the end of the each chapter to avoid any discrepancy and inconvenience. Although every effort has been made to verify the answers to the questions, certain inaccuracies might have crept in due to oversight/computer typographical error, I apologise for the same. I am confident that the book will serve the purpose.

Last but not the least I express my appreciation for our dynamic and most efficient member of the Presidential Body of Himalayan Institute Hospital Trust, Shri Vijay Dhasmana who has always encouraged me to write a valuable book.

I owe gratitude to my senior colleagues namely Prof. U.C. Sharma, Prof. R. Chandra, Prof. V.K.

Srivastava, Prof. (Emeritus) K.J.B.S. Gaur, Prof. P. Dayal, Prof. A. K. Lal, Prof. A. Indrayan, Prof. V.M. Gupta, Prof. B.D. Bhatia, Prof. S.C. Mohapatra, Prof. K.N.S. Yadava, Prof. V.K. Singh and Prof. R.N. Mishra.

Thanks to my colleagues Dr. C.M. Pandey, Dr. K.K. Singh, Dr. C.P. Mishra, Dr. S.P. Singh, Dr. Sanjoy Das, Dr. Sanjeev Mittal, Dr. Rahul Bansal, Dr. S. Kishor, Dr. S.D. Kandpal, Dr. C.M.S. Rawat and Dr. Ashish Verma for their valuable suggestions.

Finally, thanks are due to Mr. Pawaninder P. Vij, Director, M/s Peepee Publishers and Distributors (P) Ltd. for commissioning this project and handling its publication efficiently.

K.S. Negi

Contents

Part-I Biostatistics

Part-II Epidemiology

Part-I
Biostatistics

one

Variables, Measurement Scales and Graphs

1. Which is the following is not a discrete variable?
- **A.** Blood pressure
- **B.** Skin color
- **C.** Weight
- **D.** Patients in a ward

2. Which of the following is not a continuous variable?
- **A.** Height
- **B.** Weight
- **C.** Temperature
- **D.** Parity

3. All of the following are examples of discrete data *except:*
- **A.** Number of children in a family
- **B.** Number of patients in a hospital
- **C.** Temperature recorded at meterology department
- **D.** Parity of 100 women in a village

4. Which of the following is not an example of continuous data?
- **A.** Heights of 100 medical students
- **B.** Lifetimes of television tubes
- **C.** Marital status of university professors
- **D.** Weights of 20 TB patients

---

1 C **2 D** **3 C** **4 C**

5. **When variables are not measurable, which of the following is used to be represented?**
   A. Nominal B. Ordinal
   C. Interval D. Ratio

6. **When frequency of a variable is given in form of mild, moderate and severe, the data scale used is:**
   A. Nominal B. Ordinal
   C. Interval D. Ratio

7. **All of the following are examples of nominal scale *except:***
   A. Sex
   B. Marital status
   C. Religion
   D. Socio-economic status

8. **The scale used in measuring presence or absence of risk factor is:**
   A. Nominal B. Ordinal
   C. Interval D. Ratio

9. **Which of the following is a ratio scale?**
   A. Rank in class
   B. Height
   C. Temperature in °F
   D. Age

10. **All of the following are examples of ratio scale *except:***
    A. Grade of malnutrition
    B. Duration of hospital stay
    C. Height
    D. Weight

11. **The scale used in measuring serum creatinine (mg/dl) is:**
    A. Nominal
    B. Ordinal
    C. Interval
    D. None of the above

5 A 6 B 7 D 8 A 9 B 10 A
11 C

12. Which of the following is an interval scale?
- **A.** Apgar score
- **B.** Site of malignancy
- **C.** Body temperature
- **D.** Duration of hospital stay

13. In which of the following, sex composition can be demonstrated:
- **A.** Bar chart
- **B.** Histogram
- **C.** Pictogram
- **D.** Pie chart

14. Which of the following is not an example of compressed data?
- **A.** Frequency distribution
- **B.** Histogram
- **C.** Ogive
- **D.** Data array

15. Line diagram is used to show:
- **A.** Relationship between two variables
- **B.** Frequency distribution
- **C.** Trend of events with passage of time
- **D.** Most commonly occurring value

16. A scatter diagram indicates:
- **A.** Trend over time
- **B.** Correlation between two variables
- **C.** No relationship between variables
- **D.** Frequency of occurrence of events

17. The percentage age is depicted by:
- **A.** Bar diagram
- **B.** Histogram
- **C.** Pie chart
- **D.** Pictogram

18. A graph of a cumulative frequency distribution is called:
- **A.** Line graph
- **B.** Fractional distribution curve
- **C.** Ogive
- **D.** None of the above

---

12 C **13 A** **14 D** **15 C** **16 B** **17 C**
18 C

19. Frequency curve is obtained by smoothing:

A. Bar diagram
B. Histogram
C. Frequency polygon
D. Ogive

20. Best way to study relationship between two variables is:

A. Bar chart
B. Histogram
C. Pie chart
D. Scatter diagram

21. Which of the following is closest in meaning to variable used in statistics?

A. Quantity
B. Observation
C. Characteristic
D. Subject

22. The variable which the experimental manipulates is called the:

A. Constant variable
B. Independent variable
C. Dependent variable
D. Experimental variable

23. The variable that is observed for changes is called the:

A. Independent variable
B. Dependent variable
C. Experimental variable
D. Constant

24. Which of the following is a dependent variable?

A. Cause
B. Effect
C. Relative proportion
D. Association

---

19 C 20 D 21 C 22 B 23 B 24 B

25. When the variables are non-measurable, which of the following is used to be represented?
- A. Nominal
- B. Ordinal
- C. Ratio
- D. Variation

26. Which of the following is a qualitative variable?
- A. Height of palm tree
- B. Species of snake
- C. Amount of water in a bath tub
- D. Amount of snowfall in Mussoorie on a particular day

27. Which of the following is a quantitative variable?
- A. Colour of automobiles
- B. Temperature in a city on particular day
- C. Height of tallest boy in class
- D. Speed of travel

28. Which of the following represents a nominal scale?
- A. Temperature of water
- B. Density of the atmosphere at various levels
- C. Relative humidity
- D. Type of vegetable in a region

29. Which of the following represents an ordinal scale?
- A. Brand of shoes
- B. Telephone number
- C. Rating of emotional stability
- D. Price of shares of stock on stock exchange

30. All of the following belong to ratio scale, *except:*
- A. Number of cigarettes smoked in a day
- B. APGAR score
- C. Room temperature
- D. Duration of journey in a space

25 D **26 B** **27 C** **28 D** **29 C** **30 B**

31. Which of the following represents continuous measurement?

A. Size of family unit
B. Weight of elephant
C. Number of hits in a baseball game
D. Gender

32. A pictorial diagram of frequency distribution is:

A. Pictogram **B.** Bar diagram
C. Histogram **D.** Pie diaram

33. Which of the following is true for line diagram?

A. Ratio chart **B.** Pictogram
C. Scatter diagram **D.** Ogive

34. All of the following are charts and diagrams, *except:*

A. Frequency polygon
B. Pie chart
C. Ogive
D. Frequency distribution

35. Which of the following diagram represents a homogeneous data?

A. Curvilinear curve
B. Normal curve
C. Right skewed curve
D. Left skewed curve

36. Continuous quantitative data is analyzed by:

A. Histogram
B. Pictogram
C. Pie diagram
D. None of the above

37. All of the following are methods of presentation of medical data, *except:*

A. Normal curve
B. Frequency polygon
C. Ratio chart
D. Ogive

---

31 C **32 C** **33 A** **34 D** **35 B** **36 C**
37 A

38. A histogram is a kind of:
A. Table
B. Frequency count
C. Graph
D. Centile rank

39. Total area in the histogram is equal to:
A. Unit area
B. Total frequency
C. Zero
D. None of the above

40. In which kind of graph are points plotted over the mid-points of class intervals?
A. The bar diagram
B. The ogive
C. The frequency polygon
D. The histogram

41. The total area under the frequency polygon is:
A. One
B. $N = \sum f$
C. $N - 1$
D. Zero

42. The pattern of food and nutrient intakes is well depicted by:
A. Bar diagram
B. Histogram
C. Line diagram
D. Pie chart

43. Expectations of life at birth over periods of time is graphically presented by:
A. Frequency curve
B. Cumulative frequency curve
C. Histogram
D. Line diagram

44. In which graph is it necessary to bring the curve down to the X-axis at each end?
A. Frequency polygon
B. Histogram
C. Ogive
D. None of the above

45. The best graph for qualitative data is the:
A. Bar diagram
B. Histogram
C. Frequency polygon
D. Polyconic projection

---

38 C **39 B** **40 C** **41 B** **42 C** **43 D**
44 A **45 A**

46. Which graph consists of a series of rectangles?
- A. The cumulative frequency distribution
- B. The histogram
- C. Frequency polygon
- D. Relative frequency distribution

47. Which of the following graphs may be constructed to show relative frequency?
- A. Histogram
- B. Bar diagram
- C. Frequency polygon
- D. All of the above

48. Percentages of calories derived from foods of animal and vegetable origin are depicted by:
- A. Pie diagram
- B. Bar charts
- C. Frequency curves
- D. Pictograms

49. In constructing a frequency polygon, the frequency for the interval 30-39 would be plotted at:
- A. 29.5
- B. 34.5
- C. 34
- D. 39.5

50. The cumulative graph tends to form an S-shaped figure when the uncumulated distribution has:
- A. More scores at the lower end
- B. More scores at the higher end
- C. More scores in the middle than at the ends
- D. An even distribution of scores

51. In comparing two or more frequency distributions with different numbers of cases, the preferred graph is the:
- A. Histogram
- B. Relative frequency polygon
- C. Frequency polygon
- D. Ogive

46 B 47 D 48 A 49 B 50 C 51 B

Biostatistics

two

Measures of Central Tendency

1. Which of the following can be easily determined from an Ogive?

A. Mean
B. Median
C. Mode
D. None of the above

2. In statistics, the term population is referred to:

A. Number B. People
C. Observations D. Variables

3. All are advantages of Questionnaire method of data collection *except:*

A. Simple
B. Very economic
C. Interviewer not required
D. High response rate

4. Most satisfactory method of data collection is:

A. Oral questionnaire
B. Postal questionnaire
C. Results of experiments
D. Reports and records

5. Letter grade in a statistics would be considered as:

A. A quantitative variable
B. A qualitative variable
C. A normal variable
D. A numerically scaled variable

1 B 2 C 3 D 4 A 5 A

6. The score limits of an interval are 40-43. The width of the interval is:

A. 3 B. 4
C. 4.5 D. 5

7. The exact limits of the interval (10-14) are:

A. 9.0-15.0 B. 10.0-14.5
C. 9.5-14.5 D. 9.5-13.5

8. The true limits of 9.0 are:

A. 8.95 – 9.05 B. 8.5 – 9.5
C. 8.0 – 10.0 D. 9.0 – 9.1

9. A relative frequency distribution presents frequencies in terms of:

A. Whole number
B. Fractions
C. Percentages
D. Both B and C

10. F/N gives:

A. Average frequency
B. Cumulative frequency
C. Relative frequency
D. Cumulative percenage frequency

11. Which of the following is an example of a parameter?

A. $\bar{X}$ B. n
C. μ D. None of the above

12. A population characteristics is known as:

A. A parameter
B. An element
C. A statistic
D. Numeric value

13. The sample mean, $\bar{X}$ is:

A. Always equal to the population mean
B. Never equal to the population mean
C. A statistic
D. A parameter

6 B 7 C 8 A 9 D 10 C 11 C
12 A 13 C

14. How does the computation of a sample variance differ from the computation of population variahce?

A. m is replaced by $\overline{X}$
B. N is replaced by n – 1
C. N is replaced by n
D. Both A and B

15. All the following are measures of central tendency, *except:*

A. Mean
B. Median
C. Mean deviation
D. Geometric mean

16. Central value of a set of data is termed as:

A. Mean
B. Median
C. Mode
D. Geometric mean

17. The median of a set of numbers 4, 5, 8, 6, 3, 4, 8, 10, 8, is:

A. 3
B. 6
C. 4.5
D. 28

18. The median of a set of numbers 5, 5, 12, 15, 18, 11, 7, 9 is:

A. 4
B. 33 ÷ 2
C. 41
D. 10

19. In taking median value of given data, it is assumed as:

A. Median value is most frequent value
B. Median value lies at mid point in all class intervals
C. All class intervals are of equal distribution
D. Distribution of all values in a given class interval is Uniform

20. For grouped data the median is calculated by:

A. $L_m + N/2 + \Sigma Cf \div f_m$
B. $N/2 + \Sigma Cf_m - f_m$
C. $Lm + \dfrac{N/2 - Cfm}{fm} \times i$
D. $\Sigma Cf/2 - f_m$

---

14 D 15 C 16 B 17 B 18 D 19 B
20 C

21. Median is almost equivalent to:
A. 50th percentile
B. 100th percentile
C. 75th percentile
D. 25th percentile

22. Central value of a set of 240 values can be obtained by:
A. 3rd quartile
B. 25th percentile
C. 2nd quartile
D. 6th quartile

23. For a group of n =120 subjects, 40th percentile will be:
A. 48th value
B. 40th value
C. 30th value
D. None of the above

24. If 20th percentile of weight of 200 boys of age 5 years is 18 kg then it means that:
A. 40 boys have weight less than 18 kg
B. 160 boys have weight more than 18 kg
C. 20 boys have weight less than 18 kg
D. 180 boys have weight more than 18 kg

25. The most frequently occurring value in a data is:
A. Mean
B. Mode
C. Median
D. Standard deviation

26. The mode value of the set 3, 5, 7, 9, 11 is:
A. NO mode
B. 0
C. 11
D. 5

27. The mode value(s) in the set 2, 2, 3, 3, 3, 5, 9, 10, 11, 10, 12, 10 is:
A. 12
B. 3
C. 10
D. 3 and 10

28. Geometric Mean (GM) is calculated by:
A. $x_1 x_2 x_3 \ldots x_n$
B. $\sum x_n \div n$
C. $\sqrt{\sum x_n}$
D. $\sqrt[n]{x_1 x_2 \ldots\ldots x_n}$

21 A	**22 C**	**23 A**	**24 B**	**25 B**	**26 A**
27 D	**28 D**				

29. The GM of the numbers 8, 4, 2 is:

A. 8
B. 4
C. 14 ÷ 3
D. 84

30. The Harmonic Mean (HM) is calculated by:

A. $HM = 1/\Sigma x$

B. $1/HM = \Sigma \frac{1}{x_n}$

C. $HM = 1/N \Sigma 1/x_n$

D. $1/H = 1/x_1 + 1/x_2 + \ldots 1/x_n$

31. The HM of the set 2, 4, 8 is:

A. 7/8
B. 1/14
C. 3.4
D. 3/8

32. Which of the following relationship is correct?

A. $X > GM < HM$
B. $X < GM > HM$
C. $X \geq GM \geq HM$
D. $HM - GM = X$

33. Which of the following is not a measure of central tendency?

A. P_{50}
B. Mode
C. Geometric mean
D. Mean deviation

34. In microbiology, the average dilution titers is computed by:

A. Arithmetic mean
B. Geometric mean
C. Harmonic mean
D. Median

35. The formula used in Geometric Mean is:

A. $\bar{X} = \frac{x_1 + x_2 + \ldots + x_n}{n}$

B. $\bar{X}g = \frac{n_1x_1 + n_2x_2 + \ldots + Nx_n}{n_1 + n_2 + \ldots + N}$

C. $\bar{X}g = \sqrt[n]{x_1x_2\ldots\ldots x_n}$

D. $GM = N/\Sigma\ 1/X$

---

29 B 30 B 31 C 32 C 33 D 34 B
35 C

36. The highest point of a frequency curve is most closely associated with:

A. The Mean
B. The Mode
C. The Median
D. The Geometric Mean

37. If mean, median and mode are 10, 16 and 22 respectively, the distribution is:

A. Symmetric
B. Normal
C. Positively skewed
D. Negatively skewed

38. If mean > median > mode, then the distribution is:

A. Normal
B. Positively skewed
C. Negatively skewed
D. None of the above

39. Median is preferred to mean when:

A. Population is large enough
B. Low variance is seen
C. Skewed distribution is seen
D. None of the above

40. All of the following relationships are true, *except:*

A. Mean – Mode = 3 (Mean – Median)
B. $GM = \sqrt{AM \times HM}$
C. $AM^2 + HM^2 = GM^2$
D. $\text{Skewness} = \dfrac{\text{Mean} - \text{Mode}}{\text{SD}}$

41. When AM and HM of three numbers are 14/3 and 24/7 respectively then GM is:

A. 16
B. 4
C. 2
D. None of the above

36 B 37 D 38 B 39 A 40 C 41 B

42. If AM = 25 and GM = 15 then HM is:

A. 25 B. 5
C. 9 D. 15

43. The central tendency is closely associated with:

A. Tendency of scores to cluster about the centre
B. Spread
C. Location
D. Tendency of centralizing scores

44. If one top most score in a distribution is tripled which measure will change?

A. Mean
B. Median
C. Mode
D. All of the above

45. Which measure of central tendency can take two values for a given distribution?

A. The median
B. The mode
C. The mean
D. None of the above

46. The median of scores 2, 6, 3, 8, 1, 10 is:

A. 4.5 B. 5
C. 11 D. 6

47. Balance point: Highest point of curve: Half of area as:

A. Median : Mean : Mode
B. Mode : Mean : Median
C. Mean : Median : Mode
D. Mean : Mode : Median

48. Cumulative frequency is most closely associated with:

A. Mean
B. Median
C. Mode
D. Standard deviation

---

42 C **43 C** **44 C** **45 A** **46 A** **47 D**
48 B

49. The correct formula for calculation of mode value with grouped data is:

A. Lm + N/2 – Cfm

B. $Lm - \dfrac{fm - f_1}{fm - f_1 - f_2}$

C. $Lm + \dfrac{fm - f_1}{2fm - f_1 - f_2} \times i$

D. $Lm + \dfrac{2fm}{f_1 - f_2}$

50. Which of the following is crude formula for mode?

A. Mode = 3 Mean - Median

B. Mode = 3 Mean – 2 Median

C. Mode = 2 (Mean + Median)

D. Mode = 3 Median – 2 Mean

51. If mean and median of a grouped data are 16 and 30 respectively then mode values is:

A. 18

B. 58

C. 0

D. 92

52. Incubation period of measles can be estimated by:

A. Mean

B. Mode

C. Median

D. None of the above

53. Average dental caries prevalence among different school children is described by:

A. Mode

B. Mean

C. Median

D. Geometric Mean

49 C 50 D 51 B 52 B 53 A

Biostatistics

three

Measures of Variability (or Unpredictability)

1. **In a statistical analysis, dispersion of data is measured by:**
   A. Geometric Mean B. Arithmetic Mean
   C. Mode D. Rage

2. **Which of the following is commonly used as measure of dispersion?**
   A. Mean deviation
   B. Standard deviation
   C. Range
   D. Quartile deviation

3. **Which measure is not dependent on the value of each score?**
   A. Mean
   B. Variance
   C. Standard deviation
   D. Range

4. **All are measures of dispersion *except:***
   A. Range
   B. Mean deviation
   C. Standard deviation
   D. Median

5. **Which of the following is called semi-interquartile range?**
   A. $Q_1 - Q_3$ B. $Q_2 - Q_1$
   C. $1/2\ (Q_1 + Q_3)$ D. $1/2\ (Q_3 - Q_1)$

1 D 2 B 3 D 4 D 5 D

6. Which of the following is called Inter-quartile range?

A. Highest value – lowest value
B. $Q_1 - Q_2$
C. $Q_3 - Q_1$
D. $Q_2 - Q_3$

7. The ratio of 3: 1 is achieved by:

A. Quartile
B. Third Quartile
C. Median
D. Range

8. Which of the following is an example of a distance measure?

A. Range
B. Interquartile range
C. Interfractile range
D. All the above

9. The coefficient of Quartile variation is:

A. $Q_1 - Q_2$
B. $Q_2 - Q_3/N$
C. $Q_1 - Q_3$
D. $\dfrac{Q_3 - Q_1}{Q_1 + Q_2}$

10. Which of the following is an example of a relative measure of dispersion?

A. Variance
B. Mean deviation
C. Standard deviation
D. Coefficient of variation

11. Which of the following is called quartile deviation?

A. $P_{75} - P_{25}$
B. $Q_1 - Q_3$
C. $1/2\ (Q_3 - Q_1)$
D. $\dfrac{Q_3 - Q_1}{Q_2}$

6 C 7 B 8 D 9 D 10 D 11 C

12. A percentile is calculated as:

A. $\dfrac{\text{Number of scores less than a given score}}{\text{Total Number of scores}} \times 100$

B. Total number of scores – number of score < a given number

C. $\dfrac{\text{Number of scores greater than a given score}}{\text{Total Number of scores}} \times 100$

D. 100 – number of scores less than a given number

13. The square of the variance of a distribution is the:

A. Standard deviation
B. Mean deviation
C. Absolute dispersion
D. None of the above

14. Standard deviation is calculated by one of the following formulae:

A. $\dfrac{X - \bar{X}}{n}$ B. $\dfrac{\sqrt{\Sigma (X - \bar{X})}}{n}$

C. $\dfrac{\Sigma (\bar{X} - X)^2}{n}$ D. $\sqrt{\dfrac{\Sigma (X - \bar{X})^2}{n - 1}}$

15. 20 babies are born in a hospital on the same day. All weigh 2.5 kg each, the standard deviation is:

A. 1 B. 0
C. 2.5 D. 5

16. Quadratic mean or RMS of a set of numbers 1, 2, 3, 4, 5 is:

A. 3.3 B. 3
C. 1.7 D. 55

12 A 13 D 14 D 15 B 16 A

17. Root mean square of 1, 3, 5, 7 is:

A. 84 B. 4.6

C. 21 D. 2

18. Root mean square deviation denotes:

A. Standard error of means

B. Mean deviation

C. A standard deviation

D. All the above

19. All of the following statistics are unbiased estimators, *except:*

A. The sample mean

B. The sample variance

C. The sample proportion

D. The sample size

20. The general formula for an estimate of a variance is sum of squared deviations divided by:

A. Population size

B. Sample size

C. Degrees of freedom

D. Level of significance

21. If a sample consists of three observations, 13, 14, 15, an estimate of the population standard deviation equals as:

A. $\sqrt{2/3}$ B. Zero

C. $\sqrt{1/3}$ D. 1

22. Relative dispersion is calculated by:

A. $\bar{X}$ – Standard deviation

B. $\frac{X - \bar{X}}{n}$

C. Standard deviation ÷ $\sqrt{n}$

D. $\frac{\text{Standard deviation}}{\bar{X}} \times 100$

17 B 18 C 19 D 20 C 21 D 22 D

23. In a series of 300 boys, the mean systolic blood pressure was 120 mm of Hg and the standard deviation was found to be 10. The coefficient of variation is:

A. 25
B. 8.3%
C. 40%
D. 30%

24. Dispersion of a group of data can be graphically represented by:

A. Normal curve
B. Loreng curge
C. Curvilinear curve
D. Cumulative frequency curve

25. The peakedness of a frequency distribution curve is known as:

A. Mode
B. Skewness
C. Kurtosis
D. None of the above

26. All of the following are the types of kurtosis, *except:*

A. Lepto
B. Hecto
C. Meso
D. Platy

27. All of the following are measures of dispersion, *except:*

A. Standard error
B. Range
C. Standard deviation
D. 50th percentile

28. The semi-interquartile range is most closely related to the:

A. Mean
B. Median
C. Mode
D. None of the above

29. The properties of the standard deviation are most closely related to those of the:

A. Mean
B. Median
C. Mode
D. Range

---

23 B 24 B 25 C 26 B 27 D 28 B
29 A

30. In one score in distribution is changed to another value, it is certain that:

A. The range has changed

B. The standard deviation has changed

C. The semi-interquartile range has changed

D. Neither of the above

31. A score below the mean of its distribution has a deviation from the mean that is:

A. Negative

B. Zero

C. Positive

D. Not possible to compute

32. The sum of the positive deviations from mean is always:

A. Zero

B. The same as the sum of the negative deviations from the mean

C. A negative number

D. The balance point of the distribution

---

30 B **31 A** **32 B**

Biostatistics

four

Normal Distribution and Standard Scores (Z-values)

1. Normal curve is:

A. Symmetrical B. Asymmetrical
C. Curvilinear D. Linear

2. True about normal curve includes all *except:*

A. Bell shaped
B. Mean is zero
C. Mean and standard deviation coincide
D. Total area is one

3. Which is symmetrical in the following curves?

A. Skewed B. J–shaped
C. Bimodal D. Normal

4. In a standard normal curve, the area between one standard deviation on either side of mean will be:

A. 68% B. 75%
C. 50% D. 95%

5. Normal distribution is also known as:

A. Frequency distribution
B. Student's-t distribution
C. ANOVA
D. Gaussian distribution

6. In a normal curve, the proportion of observations that lie within three standard deviation from the mean is:

A. 68.27% B. 50.85%
C. 95.45% D. 99.73%

---

1 A 2 C 3 D 4 A 5 D 6 D

7. Limits set up on either side of mean in a normal curve is called:

A. Normal limits
B. Standard limits
C. Probability limits
D. Confidence limits

8. Which is true about Normal distribution curve:

A. Standard deviation = –1, Mean = 0
B. Mean = –1, Standard deviation = 0
C. Curve skews toward left
D. Curve skews toward right

9. In a normal curve true is:

A. Mean = Standard deviation
B. Mean = Median
C. Mean = 2 Standard deviation
D. None of the above

10. Which is not true about normal distribution curve?

A. Mean, median, and mode coincide
B. Standard deviation is one
C. Mean of the curve is 100
D. Total area of the curve is one

11. Standard deviation of 1.96 corresponds with area under normal curve:

A. 68% B. 95%
C. 99% D. 50%

12. Shape of the normal curve depends on:

A. Mean
B. Standard deviation
C. Number and Nature of observations
D. All of the above

13. When referring to a curve that tails off to the left end, it would be called:

A. Positively skewed
B. Negatively skewed
C. Symmetrical
D. Skewed right

7 D 8 A 9 B 10 C 11 B 12 D
13 B

14. Z is a measure of:

A. Mean deviation
B. Standard normal variate
C. Regression coefficient
D. Standard error of mean

15. The standard score, Z is expressed as:

A. $\frac{X-\mu}{N}$ B. $\frac{X-\mu}{\sigma}$

C. $\frac{X-\mu}{N}$ D. $\frac{(X-\mu)^2}{\sigma}$

16. If Hb level in healthy females has mean 14 gm/dl and standard deviation 1.5 gm/dl, then the Z- score for a female with Hb level 12.5 gm/dl is:

A. 12.5 B. 15.5
C. 1.0 D. 1.5

17. Assume that a population has $\mu = 100$ and $\sigma = 10$. If a particular observation has a standard score of 1, it can be concluded that:

A. Its value is 110
B. It lies between 90 and 110
C. Its value is greater than 110
D. Its value is lesser than

18. If a score is selected at random from a normal distribution, the probability that it will be between z = -1 and z = +1 is:

A. About 0.05 B. About 0.50
C. About 0.68 D. None of the above

19. If the alternative hypothesis, H_A is two sided, the operating characteristic curve of a test that $\mu = \mu_0$ is:

A. Positively skewed
B. Negatively skewed
C. U–shaped
D. Normal

14 B 15 B 16 C 17 A 18 C 19 D

20. If the mean is 110 and the median is 120, it seems likely that the:

A. Distribution is positively skewed
B. Distribution is negatively skewed
C. Distribution is bimodal
D. Mode value will fall in between 110 and 120

21. The mean score on a quiz is 5, and the standard deviation is zero. This shows that:

A. Distribution is normal
B. Distribution is bimodal
C. Range is small
D. All persons scored 5 on the quiz

22. For a positively skewed distribution:

A. Mean = Median = Mode
B. Mean > Median < Mode
C. Mean > Median > Mode
D. Mean < Median < Mode

23. The degree of skewness is measured by:

A. Mean ÷ Standard deviation

B. $\dfrac{\text{Mean} - \text{Median}}{\text{Standard deviation}}$

C. $\dfrac{3\,(\text{Mean} - \text{Median})}{\text{Standard deviation}}$

D. $\dfrac{\text{Median} + \text{Mean}}{2\ \text{Standard deviation}}$

24. A population study showed a mean glucose of 86mg/dl. in a sample of 100 persons showing normal distribution. What percentage of persons have glucose above 86 mg/dl:

A. 100%
B. 50%
C. 90%
D. 95%

20 B 21 D 22 C 23 C 24 B

25. The IQs of 200 students are distributed according to the normal curve with a mean of 125 and a Standard deviation. of 10. This understands that:
- **A.** 5% will have IQs less than115
- **B.** 50% will have IQs less than 125
- **C.** 2.5% will have IQs greater than 145
- **D.** 25% will have IQs greater than 135

26. For 99% confidence limits what is true in the following?
- **A.** Reduces 99% of values
- **B.** 2.58 of Standard error of mean
- **C.** $\bar{X}$ - 2 Standard error of mean
- **D.** $\bar{X}$ + 3 Standard deviation of mean

27. If the mean is 230 and the Standard error is ±10 then 95% confidence limits would be:
- **A.** 210 to 250
- **B.** 220 to 240
- **C.** 225 to 235
- **D.** 230 to 250

28. The statistical term for normal distribution (bell shaped curve) is:
- **A.** Lepto Kurtic
- **B.** Meso Kurtic
- **C.** Platy Kurtic
- **D.** Asymmetric

29. A finding with a mean value of 17 gm/dl and Standard deviation of 1.5 implies:
- **A.** The true value lies in between 15.5 gm/dl and 18.5 gm/dl
- **B.** The true value is between 15 gm/dl and 20 gm/dl
- **C.** In repeated determinations on the same sample 95% could be expected to fall in between14 gm/dl and 20 gm/dl
- **D.** The true value has a 5% chance of being less than 15.5 gm/dl or more than 18.5 gm/dl

25 A 26 B 27 A 28 B 29 C

30. If 95% confidence interval of TB infection in children of age group (5-10) years is 20% to 30%. The chance that the prevalence could be more than 30% is:

A. ± 1.96
B. 2.5%
C. 5%
D. None of the above

31. If Standard deviation doubles, the width of the confidence interval for the population mean will be:

A. Doubled
B. Decreased
C. Not affected
D. None of the above

32. If the Standard deviation of the population is known, the confidence interval for the population mean is based on:

A. The t–distribution
B. The Binomial distribution
C. The Normal distribution
D. The Poisson distribution

33. Confidence limits are:

A. Mean ± Standard error
B. Mean + Range
C. Mean – Median
D. Mean – Standard deviation

34. For 95% confidence limit, True is:

A. Reduces 95% of values
B. 1.96 of Standard error of mean
C. 2.58 of Standard error mean
D. 5% of Standard error of mean

35. Confidence limits can be calculated by using:

A. Mean and Range
B. Median and Standard deviation
C. Mean and Standard deviation
D. Mean and observed values

30 B 31 A 32 C 33 A 34 B 35 C

36. The degree of freedom for a confidence interval for the difference between two means when the samples are independent is:

A. $n_1 + n_2$
B. $(n_1 - 1) + (n_2 - 1)$
C. $n_1 - n_2$
D. $n_1 + n_2 - 1$

37. Which of the following is true for six-sigma limits?

A. Mean < Median < Mode
B. Mean ± 1.96 standard deviation
C. Mean ± 3 standard deviation
D. Mean > Median > Mode

38. Karl Pearson's coefficient of skewness is:

A. $\dfrac{\text{Mean} - \text{Median}}{\text{Standard deviation}}$

B. $\dfrac{\text{Mean} - \text{Mode}}{\text{Standard deviation}}$

C. $\dfrac{\text{Mean deviation}}{\text{Median}}$

D. $\dfrac{\text{Standard deviation} - \text{Mean}}{\text{Mean}}$

39. For a symmetrical distribution, the coefficient of skewness is:

A. 1
B. 0.5
C. 0
D. –1.5

40. If coefficient of skewness is zero and coefficient of kurtosis is 3, then the frequency distribution is:

A. Normal
B. Lepto Kurtic
C. Platy Kurtic
D. Positively skewed

36 B **37 C** **38 B** **39 C** **40 A**

41. The range of theoretical normal curve is:

A. Infinite
B. 4 SD
C. ± 2 SD
D. 6 SD

42. Three scores in distribution are 20, 25, 35. The Z-score equivalents to the first two are -1 and -1/2 respectively. The Z-score equivalent to the third score is:

A. Zero
B. 1
C. 1/2
D. 2

43. The mean value of a set of Z-scores is:

A. Zero
B. –1
C. 1
D. Indeterminate

44. The mean and standard deviation for a set of Z-scores are:

A. Mean and standard deviation are same in magnitude
B. Mean = 1, standard deviation = 0
C. Mean = 0, standard deviation = 1
D. Mean = 0, standard deviation = 0

41 A 42 C 43 A 44 D

Biostatistics

five

Probability (or Chance) Theory

1. If an event is unaffected by the outcome of another event, the two events are said to be:

A. Dependent B. Independent
C. Mutually exclusive D. All of the above

2. Which of the following can not be a probability?

A. 1 B. 1.02
C. 0.5 D. 0.001

3. The number of ways one can obtain two heads out of three flips of a coin is:

A. One B. Two
C. Three D. Four

4. If probability of being Rh negative is 1/10, then of being Rh positive will be:

A. 1/10 B. 9/10
C. 1/2 D. 1

5. Suppose the possibility of passing a thalassaemia trait by the affected parents to children is 25%. They plan to have two children. What is the probability that both children will be thalassaemic?

A. 0.5 B. 0.75
C. 0.0625 D. 0.25

6. The probability of a value falling outside 95% confidence limit is:

A. 1 in 5 B. 1 in 15
C. 1 in 20 D. 1 in 30

1 B 2 B 3 C 4 B 5 C 6 C

7. **What is the probability that a value chosen at random from a particular population is larger than the median of the population?**
   A. 0.25 B. 0.5
   C. 1 D. 0.67

8. **Suppose that P (A) = 0.5, P (B) = 0.2, and P (A and B) = 0.2. Which of the following is true?**
   A. A and B are mutually exclusive independent
   B. A and B are mutually exclusive but not independent
   C. A and B are independent but not mutually exclusive
   D. A and B are neither independent nor mutually exclusive

9. **If A and B are mutually exclusive and exhaustive then; p (A and B):**
   A. 1
   B. Zero
   B. p (A) + p (B)
   C. p (A) + p (B) – p (A and B)

10. **Probabilities vary between:**
    A. 0 and 2 B. 0 and 100
    C. –1 and 0 D. 0 and 1

11. **Which of the following are examples of mutually exclusive events?**
    A. Snow and a temperature of 10°C
    B. Rain and a cloudless sky
    C. Walking and running at the same time
    D. All of the above

12. **Which of the following values of p represents the strongest effect?**
    A. p = 0.50 B. p = 0.75
    C. p = 0.20 D. p = 0.95

13. **p–value equal to 0.33 means that the event:**
    A. Has about one chance is three of occurring
    B. Has about 3 chances in 1000 of occurring
    C. Has about 33 chances in 50 of occurring
    D. Is very unlikely to occur

---

7 B 8 D 9 B 10 D 11 D 12 C
13 A

14. The probability of an impossible event is:

A. 1 **B.** 0.5
C. 0 **D.** 0.01

15. Mutually exclusive events are:

A. Never dependent
B. Never independent
C. Always independent
D. Depending on each other

16. If an event has 95 chances out of 100 of occurring, the associated probability is:

A. 0.5 **B.** 0.0095
C. 0.95 **D.** 0.095

17. If probability of new born being Rh negative is 0.3, then the probability of new born being Rh positive is:

A. 0.5 **B.** 0.3
C. 0.7 **D.** 1

18. If the probability of new born being female is 0.5, then the probability of new born being male is:

A. 0.5
B. 1
C. 0
D. None of the above

19. If probability of getting Rh +ve is 0.9 and probability of new born being male is 0.5, then the probability of new born being a male with Rh –ve is:

A. 1 **B.** 0.45
C. 0.4 **D.** 0.5

20. If a person calculated p-value equal to 1.58, what does it mean?

A. The probability of an event is very high
B. An error has been made
C. The probability of an event is very low
D. The probability of the event is about 1.6 in 2

---

14 C 15 C 16 C 17 C 18 A 19 B
20 B

21. A p-value equal to 0.33 means that the event:
- **A.** Has about 33 chances in 100 of occurring
- **B.** Is very unlikely to occur
- **C.** Has one chance in 3 of occurring
- **D.** Has about 33 chances in 67 of occurring

22. If p = 0.53, the chances that the event will occur are:
- **A.** 53 per 1000
- **B.** Almost 1 in 1000
- **C.** 53 per 100
- **D.** 47 per 100

23. If the number of events favouring A is 30 and the number of favouring non-A is 90, then P(A) is:
- **A.** 0.4
- **B.** 0.25
- **C.** 0.33
- **D.** 0.05

24. If the number of events favouring non-A is 60, then P(A) is:
- **A.** 0.4
- **B.** 0.6
- **C.** 0.2
- **D.** 0.5

25. If the number of events favouring B is 55 and the number of favouring non-B is 45, then P(non-B) is:
- **A.** 1.22
- **B.** 0.45
- **C.** 0.55
- **D.** 0.01

26. Which of the following examples where the distribution' of numbers does not follow the Poison probability law?
- **A.** Telephone calls occurring in a certain time period
- **B.** Pulse rate of healthy male adults
- **C.** Erythrocytes on the individual fields of a counting chamber
- **D.** Daily emergency hospital admissions

21 C **22 C** **23 B** **24 A** **25 B** **26 B**

Biostatistics

six

Correlation and Regression

1. An association between two variables can be known by calculating:

A. Coefficient of correlation
B. Coefficient of regression
C. Standard error of mean
D. Standard deviation

2. Coefficient of correlation tends to lie between:

A. 0 to +1
B. –1 to 0
C. –1 to +1
D. –1.1 to +1.1

3. Height for weight for boys in a class is:

A. Association   B. Index
C. Proportion   D. Correlation

4. If r = -1 what does it mean:

A. Weak correlation
B. NO correlation
C. Perfect negative correlation
D. Wrong calculation

5. The correlation between triglyceride level and haemoglobin level is 0.3. What does it indicate?

A. Strong correlation
B. Weak correlation
C. Moderate correlation
D. None of the above

1 A   2 C   3 D   4 C   5 B

6. **If r = 1.02 what does it indicate:**
   A. Very strong +ve correlation
   B. Moderately +ve correlation
   C. Weak correlation
   D. Calculation of 'r' is wrong

7. **Not true about correlation coefficient 'r' is:**
   A. Tells about risk of the disease
   B. –1 correlation shows linear relationship
   C. Tells association between two variables
   D. Does not tell about causation

8. **If coefficient of correlation between height and weight is 2.2. What does it mean?**
   A. Positive correlation
   B. Negative correlation
   C. No association
   D. Wrong calculation

9. **If the correlation between height and weight is very strong. What will be the coefficient of correlation?**
   A. >1 B. <1
   C. +1.0 D. –1.0

10. **A correlation between two variables measures the degree to which they are:**
   A. Mutually exclusive
   B. Casually related
   C. Positively skewed
   D. Associated

11. **The correct formula for calculating 'r' is:**
   A. $\frac{\Sigma dx - \Sigma dy}{\Sigma dx^2}$ B. $\frac{\Sigma dx\, dy}{\sqrt{\Sigma dx^2\, \Sigma dy^2}}$
   C. $\frac{\Sigma dx^2}{N} - \frac{\Sigma dy^2}{N}$ D. $\frac{\Sigma dx - \Sigma dy}{\Sigma dy}$

6 D 7 D 8 D 9 C 10 D 11 B

12. Formula for Rank Correlation Coefficient 'ρ' is:

A. $\frac{1 + \Sigma D^2}{n^2 - 1}$ B. $1 - \Sigma D^2/N$

C. $1 - \frac{6\Sigma D^2}{n(n^2 - 1)}$ D. $1 - \Sigma D^2$

13. If $\frac{6\Sigma D^2}{n(n^2 - 1)}$ is zero, ρ(rho) is:

A. 0.00 B. +1.00

C. Highly negative D. Highly positive

14. If Σdx dy is zero, the correlation is:

A. Low negative B. High negative

C. Low positive D. None of the above

15. ρ(Rho) is used:

A. When one or both variables are only of ordinal scaling

B. When both variables are of interval or ratio scaling

C. When the data is non-linear

D. When both variables are dicotomous

16. The square of the correlation coefficient, the r^2 value represents:

A. The strength of the association between two variables

B. The risk ratio between two variables

C. The covariance of x and y

D. None of the above

17. The regression of Y on X:

A. Predicts X given Y

B. Predicts Y given X

C. Predicts Y given Y^{l}

D. Predicts X^{l} given X

12 C 13 B 14 D 15 A 16 A 17 B

18. Relationship between height Y, and age, X is given by the equation of Y = aX + b. If the curve is drawn what will be the shape?

A. Straight line
B. Positively skewed curve
C. Normal
D. Curvilinear

19. In the equation Y= aX + b, the positive relationship is considered when:

A. 'a' is negative
B. 'b' must be positive
C. 'b' must be negative
D. 'a' is positive

20. In a negative relationship (Y = aX + b):

A. 'b' must be negative
B. 'a' is negative
C. 'b' is negative
D. 'a' can be either positive or negative

21. In a perfect relationship:

A. All the points fall on the line, Y = aX + b
B. Same of the points fall on the line
C. The points form an elipse around the line
D. None of the points fall on the line

22. In an imperfect relationship:

A. All the points fall on the line
B. A relationship exists but all the points do not fall on the line
C. No relationship exists
D. A relationship exists but none of the points can fall on the line

23. If we know the value of one variable in an individual case and wish to know the value of another variable we calculate:

A. Coefficient of correlation
B. Coefficient of rank correlation
C. Coefficient of regression
D. Standard error of mean

---

18 A 19 D 20 B 21 A 22 B 23 C

24. A random sample of 25 observations is taken from an infinite population with a standard deviation equal to 10. The Std. dev. of the probability distribution of the sample mean equals:

A. 5 B. 10
C. 2 D. 10/25

25. In concept, the regression line is most closely related to which of the following statistical notions:

A. Mean B. Median
C. Variance D. Standard deviation

26. The amount of regression toward the mean is least when r is:

A. Low B. Negative
C. Positive D. High

27. The amount of regression toward the mean is least when 'r' is:

A. Zero B. Negative
C. Positive D. High

28. The regression of X on Y:

A. Predicts X given Y
B. Predicts $\bar{Y}$ given $\bar{X}$
C. Predicts Y given X
D. Predicts $\bar{X}$ given $\bar{Y}$

29. Which value of 'r' permits the greatest accuracy of prediction?

A. –0.85 B. –0.25
C. 0.50 D. 0.75

30. Systolic BP = a + b (Age) + c (BMI) is an example of:

A. Simple linear regression
B. Multiple linear regression
C. Simple curvilinear regression
D. Multiple curvilinear regression

---

24 C 25 A 26 D 27 D 28 A 29 A
30 B

31. Systolic BP (mm Hg) = 110 + 0.5 (20 < Age ≤ 60 years) is an equation which indicates:
A. Simple linear regression
B. Multiple linear regression
C. Simple curvilinear regression
D. Multiple curvilinear regression

32. The statistical method most likely used to determine the slope is:
A. Simple linear regression
B. Multiple regression
C. Logistic regression
D. Correlation

33. The amount of regression towards the mean is least when 'r' is:
A. Low
B. Negative
C. Positive
D. High

34. In which case does the regression equation predict that $Y^{I} = \bar{Y}$ for every value of X?
A. $r < 0$
B. $r = 0$
C. $r > 0$
D. None of the above

35. Coefficient of determination is defined as:
A. r = difference between two variances ÷ total variance
B. $r = 1 - \sigma/\sqrt{n}$
C. $r^2 = \frac{\text{Explained variance}}{\text{Total variance}}$
D. $r^2 = 1 - \frac{\sigma_1 - \sigma_2}{n(n^2 - 1)}$

36. Which of the following is not true for the coefficient of non-determination?
A. r^2
B. $1 - r^2$
C. $100 - r^2$
D. $1 - \rho^2 = K^2$

31 A 32 A 33 D 34 A 35 C 36 A

seven

Sampling Theory and Statistical Estimation

1. **Standard Error is due to:**
   - A. Observer error
   - B. Instrumental error
   - C. Sampling error
   - D. Conceptual error

2. **The correct formula for the standard error of the mean is:**
   - A. σ^2/n
   - B. σ/n
   - C. $\sigma/\sqrt{n}$
   - D. $\sqrt{\sigma/n}$

3. **Standard Error of means is calculated from:**
   - A. Standard. deviation of observations
   - B. Standard. deviation of means
   - C. Z – deviate
   - D. None of the above

4. **Mean is 25, variables are 100 and standard deviation is 1. What will be standard error of mean?**
   - A. 0.1
   - B. 0.01
   - C. 1
   - D. 10

5. **Mean of 400 observations is 100 and standard deviation is 8. What will be standard error of deviation?**
   - A. 0.4
   - B. 1.0
   - C. 2.0
   - D. 4.0

---

1 C 2 C 3 B 4 A 5 A

6. $\sqrt{\frac{pq}{n}}$ **indicates:**
   - **A.** Standard error of mean
   - **B.** Standard error of proportion
   - **C.** Standard error of differences in means
   - **D.** Standard error of differences in proportions

7. **When N is large, the finite population correction factor is approximately equal to**
   - **A.** 1 + n/N
   - **B.** √ 1 + n/N
   - **C.** √ N - N/n
   - **D.** √ 1 - n/N

8. **If the sample size is multiplied by 100, the Standard error of the sample mean is:**
   - **A.** Multiplied by 100
   - **B.** Divided by 100
   - **C.** Divided by 10
   - **D.** Unaffected

9. **Sampling error is classified as:**
   - **A.** α-error
   - **B.** β-error
   - **C.** γ-error
   - **D.** δ-error

10. **While calculating the incubation period for measles in a group of 36 children, the standard deviation is 3 and the mean incubation period of 9 days. The standard error will be:**
    - **A.** 0.4
    - **B.** 1
    - **C.** 0.5
    - **D.** 2

11. $\sqrt{\frac{p_1 q_1}{n_1} + \frac{p_2 q_2}{n_2}}$ **is a measure of:**
    - **A.** Standard error of difference of means
    - **B.** Standard error of difference between two proportions
    - **C.** Standard deviation of two proportions
    - **D.** Standard error of two means

12. **The standard error of prediction is a kind of:**
    - **A.** Mean
    - **B.** Median
    - **C.** Standard deviation
    - **D.** None of the above

---

6 B 7 D 8 C 9 A 10 C 11 B
12 C

13. The standard error of prediction measures variability of:

A. Predicted scores about the mean

B. Predicted scores about the regression line

C. Obtained scores about the regression line

D. Obtained scores about the mean

14. In gathering samples of a specific population, the error comes each times when the sampling was done. The cause may be:

A. Error in taking samples

B. Standard error

C. Sampling error

D. Non sampling error

15. The formula for the standard error of the difference between two means (independent samples) is:

A. $\dfrac{\sigma_1 + \sigma_2}{\sqrt{n_1 + n_2}}$ **B.** $\dfrac{\sigma_1^2 - \sigma_2^2}{n_1 + n_2}$

C. $\dfrac{\sigma_1^2}{n_1} - \dfrac{\sigma_2^2}{n_2}$ **D.** $\sqrt{\dfrac{\sigma_1^2}{n_1} + \dfrac{\sigma_2^2}{n_2}}$

16. In statistics, the precision is measured by the formula:

A. $\bar{X} - m$ **B.** $\sigma/\bar{X}$

C. $\sigma/\sqrt{n}$ **D.** $\dfrac{\sqrt{n}}{\sigma}$

17. In Random Sampling, chance of being selected is:

A. Not same and not known

B. Same and known

C. Same and not known

D. Not same but known

18. About Random Sampling not true is:

A. Simple **B.** Biasness

C. Stratified **D.** Systematic

---

13 C **14 C** **15 D** **16 D** **17 B** **18 B**

19. True about Simple Random Sampling is:

A. Technique provides least number of possible samples
B. Every fixed unit is taken for selection
C. All units have equal chance to be selected
D. Only selected units have right to be selected

20. A sample selected by a process of chance is:

A. A large sample
B. A exact sample
C. A random sample
D. A numerical scaled sample

21. The idea of a random sample is particularly important for:

A. Measuring degree of association
B. All types of analysis
C. Descriptive statistics
D. Statistical Inference

22. For a survey, a village is divided into 5 lanes then each lane is sampled randomly. It is an example of:

A. Simple Random Sampling
B. Stratified Random Sampling
C. Systematic Random Sampling
D. Multi stage Sampling

23. Which is true of cluster sampling:

A. Every n^{th} case is chosen for study
B. Involves the use of Random Numbers
C. A natural group is taken as sampling unit
D. Stratification of population is done

24. A selection of every unit from a normally distributed population is utilizing:

A. Simple Random Sampling
B. Systematic Sampling
C. Stratified Sampling
D. Complete enumeration

---

19 C   20 C   21 D   22 B   23 C   24 D

25. The Cluster Sampling Technique used for evaluating UIP coverage is:

A. 30 cluster of 5 children
B. 30 cluster of 10 children
C. 30 cluster of 7 children
D. 20 cluster of 7 children

26. All the following are Random Sampling methods *except:*

A. Simple Random Sampling
B. Stratified Sampling
C. Cluster Sampling
D. Quota Sampling

27. The fundamental condition that permits proper statistical inference is:

A. Random sampling
B. Having a large sample
C. Normal distribution of scores
D. Knowledge of the values of parameters of the population

28. In systematic random sampling, the sample interval is determined by:

A. Population : Sample
B. Total population ÷ Sample size desired
C. $\frac{\text{Total population}}{\text{Sample}} \times 100$
D. None of the above

29. As sample size increases, standard deviation of sample means, $\sigma_{\bar{X}}$:

A. Decreases
B. Increases
C. Remains the same
D. Approaches to infinity

30. The effect size 'd' depends on:

A. Power of Test
B. Standard deviation
C. Level of significance
D. None of the above

---

25 C **26 D** **27 A** **28 B** **29 A** **30 B**

31. For qualitative data, the sample size can be calculated by:

A. $n = \frac{2pq}{L^2}$ **B.** $n = \frac{4pq}{L}$

C. $n = \frac{4pq}{L^2}$ **D.** $n = \frac{pq}{L}$

32. For quantitative data, the sample size(n) is computed by the formula:

A. $\frac{4\sigma}{L}$ **B.** $\frac{4\sigma^2}{L^2}$

C. $\frac{2\sigma}{L^2}$ **D.** $\frac{2\sigma^2}{L}$

33. The statistical hypothesis to be tested is called the:

A. Trial hypothesis
B. Null hypothesis
C. Alternative hypothesis
D. Directional hypothesis

34. When the null hypothesis is H_0: $\mu = 40$, the alternative hypothesis, H_A can be:

A. $H_A : \mu < 40$
B. $H_A : \mu \neq 42$
C. $H_A : \mu \geq 40$
D. None of the above

35. Which could be an alternative hypothesis for a comparison of two means?

A. $\mu_1 = \mu_2$ **B.** $\mu_1 < \mu_2$
C. $\bar{X}_1 > \bar{X}_2$ **D.** $\bar{X}_1 < \bar{X}_2$

36. Which is the usual null hypothesis for a comparison of two means?

A. $\bar{X}_1 = \bar{X}_2$ **B.** $\bar{X}_1 \neq \bar{X}_2$
C. $\mu_1 = \mu_2$ **D.** $\mu_1 \neq \mu_2$

31 C 32 B 33 B 34 A 35 B 36 C

37. $H_O : H_A$ as

A. Specified in advance	: Specified later
B. True	: False
C. Accept	: Reject
D. Specific	: Non specific

38. When the results are statistically significant, this means:

A. The independent variable has a large effect

B. Rejecting null hypothesis

C. The obtained probability is equal to or less than α

D. Both B and C

39. The area of the region of acceptance expressed as a proportion of the total area under the curve is:

A. α B. $\alpha/2$

C. $1 - \alpha$ D. $1 - \alpha/2$

40. When a null hypothesis is accepted, it is possible that:

A. A correct decision has been made

B. A type I error has been made

C. Both A and B

D. None of the above

41. Statistical significance means:

A. Rejection of H_O

B. Rejection of H_A

C. A significant finding after the statistical analysis

D. An important difference between observed and expected values

42. Power of a test equals:

A. α error + β error B. $1 - \beta$ error

C. $1 - \alpha$ error D. α error – β error

43. The power of an experiment is affected by:

A. The α – level

B. sample size

C. The magnitude of the independent variable's effect

D. All of the above

37 D 38 D 39 C 40 A 41 A 42 B
43 D

44. Rejecting the null hypothesis means there may be:
A. A type I error
B. A type II error
C. A correct decision
D. Both B and C

45. A type I error is committed when a:
A. False H_O is accepted
B. True H_O is rejected
C. True H_A is accepted
D. α is higher than it should be

46. Suppose that the null hypothesis, H_o is true and it is rejected, then this is a:
A. Type I error, and its probability is α
B. Type II error, and its probability is β
C. Type I error, and its probability is β
D. Type II error, and its probability is α

47. A type II error is committed when a:
A. False H_O is accepted
B. True H_O is rejected
C. False H_A is accepted
D. α is higher than it should be

48. Which is a non directional alternative hypothesis?
A. $\bar{X} \neq 100$
B. $\mu > 100$
C. $\bar{X} < 100$
D. $\mu \neq 100$

49. Another term for a type II error is:
A. Alpha error
B. Beta error
C. Gamma error
D. None of the above

50. The 'power' in a study is best defined as:
A. An inappropriate sample size
B. Alpha error
C. Chances of making a type I error
D. Chances of making a type II error

---

44 A 45 B 46 A 47 A 48 D 49 B
50 D

51. The value of a serves as protection against:

A. Selection bias
B. Type I error
C. Type II error
D. Inadequate sample size

52. P-value is the probability of:

A. Rejecting a null hypothesis when it is true
B. Not rejecting a null hypothesis when it is true
C. Rejecting a null hypothesis when it is false
D. Not rejecting a null hypothesis when it is false

53. All of the following statements are true, *except:*

A. Sample size is necessary to achieve statistical significance
B. Sample size is essential to achieve medical significance
C. A statistically significant result may and may not be medically significant
D. Larger the sample size, more is the chance of getting statistical significance

54. Which of the following is not true about type-II error?

A. Type-II error is more serious than type-I error
B. Probability of type-II error is also called beta-error
C. Rejecting H_0 when it is true
D. Power is the complement of probability of type-II error

51 B 52 A 53 B 54 A

Biostatistics

eight

Tests of Hypotheses and Significance

1. The basic goal of hypothesis testing is:
 A. To establish the value of α
 B. To establish the value of β
 C. To confirm the alternative hypothesis
 D. To distinguish between random and meaningful differences in outcome

2. The levels of significance most commonly used are:
 A. 0.10 and 0.05
 B. 0.05 and 0.01
 C. 0.01 and 0.001
 D. 0.002 and 0.005

3. The difference between two samples is regarded as statistically significant when the p-value is:
 A. 0.5 to 0.1
 B. < 0.05
 C. 0.01 to 0.05
 D. > 0.05

4. Statistical significance is achieved when:
 A. α is greater than p
 B. $\beta = \alpha$
 C. $p > \alpha$
 D. $p > b$

5. If the out come of a test is significant at the 0.01 level, it:
 A. Will not be significant at the 0.05 level
 B. Will be also significant at the 0.05 level
 C. Will probably not be significant at any level
 D. May be significant at any level

1 D 2 B 3 B 4 A 5 B

6. Statistical significance means:

A. A significant finding, after the statistical analysis

B. A difference between observed and expected value

C. Rejection of Null hypothesis

D. Rejection of Alternative hypothesis

7. Generally 'degrees of freedom' is most closely related to:

A. The a-level

B. The sample size

C. $\overline{X}$

D. S.E. of $\overline{X}$

8. If $\alpha = 0.05$ and the probability of a type II error is 0.1457, the power of the test is:

A. 0.95

B. 0.8543

C. 1.1457

D. None of the above

9. Which of the following will not increase the power of a test?

A. Decreasing α - level

B. Increasing sample size

C. Reducing experimental error

D. Using directional hypotheses where appropriate

10. If $\alpha = 0.01$, one tailed test, which of the following one tailed p-values would lead to the rejection of H_0?

A. 0.02 **B.** 0.05

C. 0.004 **D.** 0.015

11. If $\alpha = 0.05$, two tailed test, which of the following two tailed p-values would lead to rejection of H_0?

A. p = 0.03 **B.** p = 0.06

C. p = 0.50 **D.** p = 0.10

---

6 C 7 B 8 B 9 B 10 C 11 A

12. To test the hypothesis of no difference between the means of two independent samples. The first sample consists of 30 cases and the second consists of 20 cases. The number of degrees of freedom for the test is:

A. 50 B. 10
C. 48 D. 49

13. To test the hypothesis of no difference between the means of two dependent samples. There are 30 cases in the first sample and 30 cases in the second. The number of d.f. for the test will be:

A. 58 B. 28
C. 29 D. 59

14. The contingency table is a form of:

A. Frequency distribution
B. Relative frequency distribution
C. Cumulative frequency distribution
D. Bivariate frequency distribution

15 In a contingency table, the number of degrees of freedom is:

A. Rows × Columns
B. (Rows + Columns) – 1
C. (Rows – 1) (Columns –1)
D. Rows + Columns – 2

16. The normal deviate test is used with:

A. A replicated measures design
B. A single sample design
C. A multi-group design
D. An independent groups design

18. Null hypothesis can be rejected, if:

A. Z obtained = Z critical
B. Z obtained ≥ Z critical
C. |Z obtained| ≥ |Z critical|
D. Z obtained ≤ Z critical

---

12 C 13 C 14 D 15 C 16 B 17 C
18 D

19. To use the Z-test:

A. The sampling distribution of $\bar{x}$ should be normal

B. The population of raw scores must be normally distributed

C. μ and σ must be specified

D. Both A and B

20. Which of the following is most likely to contribute to a statistically significant but clinically meaningless outcome?

A. Setting α at 0.05

B. Obtaining a p-value >0.05

C. Performing a two tailed test

D. Using a very large sample

21. The statistical procedure by which the participants are allocated into groups usually called study and control groups, is called:

A. Classification
B. Stratification
C. Randomization
D. Follow up

22. Standard drug when used 40% patients respond and when new drug was used 60% patients responded. Which of the following Tests of significance is most useful in this study?

A. Z – Test
B. χ^2 – Test
C. Student's t – Test
D. Fisher t – Test

23. The statistical analysis of two unrelated big data (n = 200 in done by:

A. Paired t – Test
B. Unpaired t – Test
C. χ^2 – Test
D. Z – Test

24. If the Standard deviation of the population is unknown, and the sample size is less than 10, the confidence interval for the population mean is based on:

A. The normal distribution

B. The t – distribution

C. The Binomial distribution

D. The Poisson distribution

19 B 20 D 21 C 22 A 23 D 24 B

25. As the number of degree of freedom increases, Student t-distribution:

A. Remains the same
B. Changes rapidly at first, then more slowly
C. Changes slowly at first, then more rapidly
D. Changes at a fixed interval

26. The mean BP of a group of patients was determined and after an investigation trial, the mean BP estimated again. The Test to be applied to determine the significance of intervention is:

A. χ^2 – Test
B. Paired t – Test
C. Correlation coefficient
D. Z – Test

27. As the degree of freedom increases, the t-distribution:

A. Approaches the normal distribution
B. Gets more symmetrical
C. Remains the same
D. Becomes more skewed

28. The mean of the t-distribution equals:

A. Zero **B.** 1
C. μ **D.** σ

29. In a Student's t-test, when the size of the sample is increased, the confidence interval:

A. Increases **B.** Decreases
C. Remains the same **D.** Changes shape

30. All of the following statements are the about non-parametric Test *except:*

A. Distribution free test is synonyms of non-parametric test
B. It is a parameter-free test is synonyms of non-parametric test
C. It is applied where the test-statistics are independent of the parameters
D. It is only applicable when quick or preliminary data analysis not needed

25 B 26 B 27 A 28 A 29 B 30 D

31. All of the following statistical tests are non-parametric *except:*

A. Chi-square Test **B.** Sign Test
C. Runs Test **D.** The Z-Test

32. The most appropriate statistical test to compare the distribution of laboratory values in men with that of women is :

A. χ^2 test **B.** Unpaired t – test
C. Correlation **D.** Regression

33. χ^2 – Value is calculated by the formula:

A. $\dfrac{O-E}{E}$ **B.** $\Sigma \dfrac{O-E}{n}$

C. $\Sigma \dfrac{(O-E)^2}{E}$ **D.** $\dfrac{\Sigma (O-E)^2}{E}$

34. In general, the number of degree of freedom for row, R by column, C interaction is giver by:

A. (R + C) – 1 **B.** (R – 1) (C – 1)
C. (R – 1) + (C – 1) **D.** R × C

35. While applying χ^2 – Test to a contingency table of three rows and three columns, the degree of freedom would be:

A. 9 **B.** 8
C. 4 **D.** 7

36. A chi-square value can never be negative because:

A. The absolute value of the differences is completed
B. Difference between observed and expected frequencies are squared
C. A negative value would mean that the observed frequencies were negative
D. None of the above

---

31 D 32 B 33 C 34 B 35 C 36 B

37. χ^2 – Test is:

A. The square root of proportion means
B. The standard deviation of proportion means
C. Not valid for value below 5
D. The difference of two means

38. The χ^2 –Test is not valid unless:

A. All the expected frequencies are greater than 5
B. Both variable are continuous
C. The sample size is large
D. At least one variable is from a normal distribution

39. X is a random variable with the χ^2- distribution. The probability that it exceeds 32.00 equals to 0.01. Its number of degree of freedom is:

A. 12 B. 14
C. 16 D. 18

40. If a random variable has a χ^2 – distribution with 7 degrees of freedom, χ^2 at 0.05 l.s. equals:

A. 12.592 B. 14.067
C. 16.919 D. Less than 14

41. Which of the following is not relate with χ^2 – Test:

A. Normal population
B. Level of significance
C. Degree of freedom
D. N < 30

42. Study that is used to compare serum cholesterol levels in obese and non-obese women, and to find the relation or significance prevalence is:

A. Paired t – Test
B. χ^2 – Test
C. Z – Test
D. Unpaired t – Test

37 C 38 A 39 C 40 B 41 D 42 B

43. An appropriate statistical method to compare two proportions is:

A. Student's t-test
B. Correlation coefficient
C. χ^2 – test
D. Sign test

44. In using the χ^2 – test for statistical analysis of a 2 × 2 contingency table, the H_0 is:

A. That the row and column totals are the same
B. That the two means do not differ
C. That p is <0.05
D. That the two variables are independent to each other

45. χ^2 is used to test difference between:

A. Proportions
B. Means
C. Variances
D. None of the above

46. χ^2 may be used with:

A. Nominal data
B. Ordinal data
C. Ratio data
D. All of the above

47. A multivariable analysis is appropriate when:

A. Multiple hypotheses are being tested
B. Multiple outcome variables are under investigation
C. Multiple repetitions of an experiment are planned
D. More than one independent variable is under investigation

48. Which of the following statements is considered a multivariate model?

A. Height and weight very together
B. Height varies with age, weight, and sex
C. Height and weight vary with age and sex
D. None of the above

43 C 44 D 45 A 46 D 47 D 48 B

49. All of the following are included in the multivariate model *except:*

A. y – intercept
B. The outcome variable
C. Degrees of freedom
D. An error term

50. What is the test – statistic used in analysis of variance?

A. Z statistic
B. F statistic
C. Chi square
D. None of the above

51. One way ANOVA is applicable when there are:

A. Any number of matched subgroups
B. Any number of independent subgroups
C. No more than five independent subgroups
D. No more than five matched subgroups

52. A variance estimate is computed from:

A. Sample differences
B. Sample means
C. Sum of squared deviations
D. Population variances

53. $\Sigma(\bar{X} - \bar{X}_T)^2$ is a measure of:

A. Total variation
A. Within-groups variation
B. Among-groups variation
C. None of above

54. $\Sigma(\bar{X} - \bar{X})^2$ is measure of:

A. Total variation
B. Within-groups variation
C. Among-groups variation
D. None of the above

55. The F distribution is:

A. The ratio between two variance estimates
B. The difference between two variance estimates
C. The difference between two sample variances
D. The ratio between two population variances

---

49 C 50 B 51 B 52 C 53 C 54 B
55 A

56. F ratio is based on:

A. df_A
B. df_T
C. Both A and B
D. None of the above

57. F-ratio is:

A. $MS_A \div MS_E$
B. $MS_W \div MS_A$
C. $SS_T - SS_A$
D. $SS_E + SS_A$

58. In a one way analysis of variance:

A. There may be any number of levels of a sample variable
B. Total sum of squares may be partitioned into only one source of variance
C. Between-group sum of squares minus within-group sum of squares equals total sum of squares
D. None of the above

59. Which of the following statements is not true about life table:

A. It is a bivariate table
B. It is a measure of vital events
C. It is used to find survival rate after treatment or operation in a chronic disease
D. It helps to project population estimates by age and sex

60. All are true about Kappa(K) statistic *except:*

A. Agreement between two observers on a binary variable
B. Ratio of sensitivity and specificity
C. $K = \dfrac{\text{Observed agreement} - \text{Chance agreement}}{1 - \text{Chance agreement}}$
D. Agreement beyond chance divided by the amount of agreement possible beyond chance

61. When H_0 is true, the expected value of F-ratio is:

A. <0
B. >0 but <1
C. = 1
D. >1

56 A 57 A 58 A 59 A 60 B 61 C

62. **The Sign test:**
   A. Specifies that each observation be given a + or – sign
   B. Uses the binomial distribution
   C. Assumes normality
   D. Both A and B

63. **The statistic used in the sign test measures:**
   A. The direction of the difference between pairs and scores
   B. The difference between the means of the two groups
   C. The magnitude of the difference between pairs and scores
   D. The difference between the variance of the two groups

64. **In the sign test, if the null hypothesis is true, then p:**
   A. Equals 0.50
   B. Is greater than 0.50
   C. Is less than 0.50
   D. Differs depending an alternative hypothesis

65. **The sign test:**
   A. Is used with a repeated measures design
   B. Analyses the sign of difference scores
   C. Uses the binomial distribution
   D. All of the above

66. **Which of the following is correct test – criterion for Z-test of proportions?**
   A. $\dfrac{p_1 - p_2}{\dfrac{p_1}{n_1} + \dfrac{p_2}{n_2}}$
   B. $\dfrac{p_1 - p_2}{\sqrt{\dfrac{p_1 q_1}{n_1} + \dfrac{p_2 q_2}{n_2}}}$
   C. $\dfrac{p_1 - p_2}{\text{S.E. of } p_1 - p_2}$
   D. $\dfrac{p_1 - p_2}{N (p_1 + p_2)}$

62 D 63 A 64 A 65 D 66 B

67. The null hypothesis in the one way analysis of variance states that:

A. All samples have the same mean
B. All populations have the same variance
C. All samples have the same variance
D. All populations have the same mean

68. If the H_0 in the one way analysis of variance is false then:

A. S_A^2 is likely to be greater than Sw^2
B. S_A^2 is likely to be about the same size as Sw^2
C. Homogeneity of variance can not occur
D. S_A^2 is likely to be smaller than Sw^2

69. The degrees of freedom for the among groups variance estimate is:

A. $k - 1$
B. $n_T - k$
C. k
D. $n_T - 1$

70. In the analysis of variance, which quantity is analyzed:

A. SS_A
B. SS_W
C. σ^2
D. SS_T

71. F-ratio is based on which of the following degrees of freedom?

A. df_A
B. df_T
C. Both A and B
D. None of the above

72. In a two way factorial analysis of variance, which of the following quantities is a part of the total sum of squared deviations?

A. SS_A
B. SS_R
C. SS_W
D. None of the above

73. Which of the following tests assumes that the populations of interest all have a normal shape?

A. The sign test
B. The run test
C. The Mann-Whitney test
D. The t – Test

---

67 D 68 A 69 A 70 D 71 A 72 B
73 D

74. A sample of scores consists of the values 88, 84, 87, 88, 89, 88, 85, 88, 90. When we rank-order these scores, the first score of 88 on the list should receive the rank of:

A. 5.5 **B.** 22
C. 1 **D.** 4

75. When there are ten or more pairs of scores, the sign test employs which of the following statistics?

A. t-test
B. Z-test
C. Chi-squaretest
D. F-ratio test

76. Which test assumes that sampling was random?

A. The sign test
B. The Mann-Whitney test
C. F-test
D. All of the above

77. The sum of a test of ranks can be found from the formula:

A. $n(n-1)/2$
B. $n(n-1)$
C. $n(n+1)/2$
D. $(n_1-1)+(n_2-1)$

74 A 75 C 76 D 77 C

Biostatistics

nine

Demography and Vital Statistics

1. **Demography includes study of all *except:***
   A. Fertility
   B. Mortality
   C. Morbidity
   D. Migration and marriages

2. **All of the following statements are related to demography *except:***
   A. Changes in population size
   B. Composition of the population
   C. Disease pattern in population
   D. Distribution of population in space

3. **All of the following statements are true for census *except:***
   A. Census is to provide demographic information
   B. It is taken in the country at regular intervals of 10 years
   C. The first regular census in India was done in 1881
   D. It is taken by primary health workers

4. **Data collected by health information system is useful for:**
   A. Measuring the health status of the people
   B. Assessing the attitudes and degree of satisfaction of the beneficiaries
   C. National and International comparison of health status
   D. All of the above

---

1 C **2 C** **3 D** **4 D**

5. Which of the following is not true about Census?

A. First regular census in India was taken in 1881
B. Usually conducted in the month of March at every tenth year
C. Computes vital statistics and other indicators
D. The full results become available in a short time

6. Population count is taken on:

A. 1st January B. 1st March
C. 1st July D. 1st April

7. All are true statements regarding sample registration system *except:*

A. Covers only certain parts of the country
B. Provides denominator for calculating rates
C. Dual record system
D. Independent survey every six months

8. Age and sex composition of population can be demonstrated by:

A. Histogram
B. Age pyramid
C. Line diagram
D. Scatter diagram

9. Yearly estimation of population is made by:

A. Arithmetic increase method
B. Geometric increase method
C. Natural increase method
D. All of the above

10. The sample registration system was started to get information on:

A. Birth and death rates for the states and country
B. Morbidity rates of various diseases for the states and country
C. Migration data from the country
D. None of the above

5 D 6 C 7 A 8 B 9 D 10 A

11. All are advantages of questionnaire method of data collection *except:*

A. Simple
B. Cheap
C. Interviewer is not required
D. High response rate

12. Hospital data are not good source of health information because of all *except:*

A. Population at risk can not be defined
B. Admission policy may differ
C. Mild cases are not attended
D. Provide only the denominator

13. For calculating literacy rate, the age group included is:

A. ≥ 5 years B. ≥ 7 years
C. ≥ 10 years D. ≥ 18 years

14. In census literacy is assessed by:

A. Schooling upto primary
B. Ability to read and write
C. Ability to write i.e., signature
D. Ability to read newspaper

15. The denominator to calculate literacy rate is:

A. Population above 14 years of age
B. Entire population
C. Population above 7 years of age
D. Population above 5 years of age

16. Family size is related to:

A. Total number of female born
B. Total number of male born
C. Total number of family members
D. Total number of children born

17. The cause of death in a village is assessed by:

A. Census
B. Sample Registration System
C. Mortality Investigation
D. Model Registration System

---

11 D 12 D 13 B 14 B 15 C 16 C
17 B

18. Percentage of population which is under 15 years of age is:

A. 15% B. 25%
C. 40% D. 60%

19. The primary function of census is:

A. To find out age and sex distribution of population
B. To find out different mortality rates
C. Population enumeration
D. To find out birth and death rates

20. Which of the following statement is true for the term 'eligible couple'?

A. A couple having two living children
B. A couple with wife in reproductive age group
C. A couple who is ready to undergo sterilization
D. A couple having three or more children

21. In India, eligible couples per 1000 population is:

A. 50 – 70 B. 100 – 150
C. 150 – 180 D. 200 – 250

22. Population pyramid is related with:

A. Age and sex composition
B. Birth - death rates
C. Morbidity and mortality pattern
D. Age wise distribution of population

23. The population of children in the age group of 0 – 6 years in the population is about:

A. 6% B. 13%
C. 20% D. 27%

24. The percentage of women to the total population of India in the reproductive age group is:

A. 16% B. 22%
C. 25% D. 35%

25. The percentage of school age children in India's population is about:

A. 15% B. 25%
C. 30% D. 40%

---

18 C **19 C** **20 B** **21 C** **22 A** **23 B**
24 B **25 B**

26. The number of children in 0–4 years of age per 1000 women of child bearing age (15-49) years is defined as:

A. Child-woman ratio
B. Gross reproduction rate
C. Total fertility rate
D. None of the above

27. For a population of 1000, a sex ratio more than 1000 means:

A. Males are less than 500
B. Females are less than 500
C. Males and females are equal
D. None of the above

28. Best single parameter for assessing physical growth is:

A. Weight for age
B. Height for age
C. Chest circumference
D. Skin fold thickness

29. Physical quality of life index in India is:

A. 31
B. 43
C. 50
D. 61

30. PQLI includes all *except:*

A. Per capital income
B. Life expectancy at age 1 year
C. Literacy
D. Infant mortality

31. Which one of the following is not a socio-economic indicator?

A. Dependency ratio
B. Literacy
C. Life expectancy at birth
D. Housing

26 A **27 A** **28 A** **29 B** **30 A** **31 C**

32. Child-woman ratio is:
A. 0 – 4 years of children and 15 – 44 years of women
B. 0 – 4 years of children and 15 – 45 years of married women
C. 0 – 4 years of children and 20 – 30 years of married women
D. 0 – 5 years of children and 18 – 21 years of women

33. Male to female ratio is:
A. Males for 1000 population
B. Females for 1000 population
C. Males for 1000 females
D. Males and females for 1000 population

34. In calculating dependency ratio, the numerator is:
A. Population less than 10 years and 60^+
B. Population < 15 years and 60^+
C. Population < 10 years and 65^+
D. Population < 15 years and 65^+

35. The average expectation of life at birth:
A. Increase with improvement of health
B. Decreases as death rate increases
C. Is higher in females than males
D. Has all the above characteristics

36. Which of the following is a dependent variable?
A. Cause
B. Effect
C. Association
D. Relative proportion

37. The most common use of life table is made by:
A. Life insurance company
B. General insurance company
C. Radar establishment in defence
D. All of the above

32 A 33 B 34 B 35 D 36 B 37 A

38. Growth pattern of a population having annual growth rate of 1.5 to 2% is:
- **A.** Slow growth
- **B.** Moderate growth
- **C.** Very rapid growth
- **D.** Explosive growth

39. If annual growth rate of population is 1.5 to 2% then it will double in:
- **A.** 28 to 23 years
- **B.** 35 to 28 years
- **C.** 47 to 35 years
- **D.** 70 to 47 years

40. Early expanding stage in demographic cycle is characterized by:
- **A.** Low birth rate, declining death rate
- **B.** Unchanged birth rate, declining death rate
- **C.** High birth rate, declining death rate
- **D.** High death rate, high birth rate

41. More declining birth rate and death rate tend to fall, the stage is:
- **A.** Early expanding
- **B.** Late expanding
- **C.** Declining
- **D.** Stationary

42. In what stage of demographic cycle in India at present?
- **A.** Low stationary
- **B.** High stationary
- **C.** Early expanding
- **D.** Late expanding

43. The year of 'Big Divide' was:
- **A.** 1901
- **B.** 1921
- **C.** 1931
- **D.** 1951

44. In demography, total fertility rate includes:
- **A.** Total number of live births in a family
- **B.** Approximate magnitude of completed family size
- **C.** Average number of female children born per 1000 women
- **D.** Number of live births per 1000 women in the age group of 15-45 years

---

38 C 39 C 40 B 41 B 42 D 43 B 44 B

45. Vital statistics deals with:
- **A.** Births and deaths
- **B.** Births, deaths and marriages
- **C.** Sickness and deaths
- **D.** Births, deaths, marriages and sickness

46. Vital statistics is collected from:
- **A.** Census
- **B.** Previous hospital records
- **C.** Epidemiological surveillance
- **D.** All of the above

47. What is the denominator in general fertility rate?
- **A.** Ever married women
- **B.** Women in reproductive age group 15 – 44 years
- **C.** Married women in the age group 15 – 44 years
- **D.** All the women

48. In defining general fertility rate the denominator is:
- **A.** Mid year population
- **B.** Number of women in 15-45 years of age group
- **C.** Number of married women
- **D.** Number of live births

49. In demography, estimated family size is given by:
- **A.** General fertility rate
- **B.** Total fertility rate
- **C.** Net reproduction rate
- **D.** General marital fertility rate

50. NRR = 1 implies a couple protection rate of:
- **A.** 50% **B.** 60%
- **C.** 90% **D.** 100%

51. The best measure of fertility pattern is:
- **A.** NRR
- **B.** GRR
- **C.** Child-woman ratio
- **D.** CBR

45 B 46 D 47 B 48 B 49 B 50 B
51 A

52. The denominator in GRR is:
- **A.** Women in the reproductive age group
- **B.** Married women
- **C.** Married women in the age group 15 – 45
- **D.** All live births

53. Fertility rate can be reduced by:
- **A.** Spacing of pregnancies
- **B.** Early marriages
- **C.** Change of MTP Act
- **D.** Compulsory sterilization

54. The demographic gap is the difference between:
- **A.** Birth and death rates
- **B.** General and Total fertility rates
- **C.** GRR and NRR
- **D.** Age specific birth and death rates

55. The median age of a population principally determined by:
- **A.** The CDR
- **B.** The age adjusted mortality rate
- **C.** The prevalence of chronic disease
- **D.** The CBR

56. For vital statistics, the population used is as on:
- **A.** 1st January
- **B.** 1st April
- **C.** 1st July
- **D.** 1st October

57. In birth and death registration act, registration of birth is done within:
- **A.** One week **B.** Two weeks
- **C.** Three weeks **D.** One month

58. Registration of death should be done within:
- **A.** 24 hours **B.** 48 hours
- **C.** 72 hours **D.** 7 days

---

52 A 53 A 54 A 55 B 56 C 57 A 58 C

59. Child survival index per 1000 births is calculated by subtracting one of the following rate from 1000:

A. Infant mortality rate
B. Neonatal mortality rate
C. Under 5 mortality rate
D. None of the above

60 The number of deaths in people aged above 50 years as a percentage of total deaths is known as:

A. Crude death rate
B. Specific death rate
C. Proportional mortality ratio
D. Expectancy of life

61. The denominator for calculating birth rate is:

A. Total number of live births
B. Number of female population
C. Mid year population
D. Number of women in reproductive age group (15-45 yrs)

62. Which of the following is a sensitive indicator of family planning achievement?

A. Abortion rate
B. General fertility rate
C. Birth rate
D. Age specific fertility rate

63. An index of fertility which takes into account the fertility and mortality situation prevailing in community is:

A. CDR **B.** TFR
C. NRR **D.** GRR

64. Child Survival Rate per 1000 live births is calculated by subtracting from 1000:

A. Infant mortality
B. Post neonatal mortality
C. Under 5 mortality
D. 1-4 years mortality

59 C 60 C 61 C 62 D 63 C 64 C

65. In maternal mortality rate, denominator is:
- **A.** All women belonging to 15 – 49 years of age
- **B.** 1000 pregnancies
- **C.** 1000 population
- **D.** 1000 live birth

66. Maternal mortality ratio in India is estimated to be:
- **A.** 0.5 per 1000 live births
- **B.** 1.5 per 1000 live births
- **C.** 4.08 per 1000 live births
- **D.** 5.5 per 1000 live births

67. Infant mortality rate includes children:
- **A.** 1-3 years of age
- **B.** Pre school children
- **C.** Still birth
- **D.** Less than 1 year of age

68. Child death rate includes deaths occurring in children:
- **A.** 1-4 years
- **B.** < 5 years
- **C.** Up to 9 years
- **D.** 1-5 years

69. The denominator is in under 5 mortality rate is:
- **A.** Total number of children aged 1-5 years
- **B.** Number of live births in the same year
- **C.** Total number of deliveries occurred in the population
- **D.** Mid year population

70. All of the following deaths are classified as maternal death *except:*
- **A.** During abortion
- **B.** During third month of lactation
- **C.** During labor
- **D.** During first 42 days after delivery

---

65 D　66 C　67 D　68 A　69 B　70 B

71. The birth and death rates are registered according to national and states survey done by 6 month is called:
- A. SRS
- B. Social Security Scheme
- C. Demographic survey
- D. Epidemiological surveillance

72. Age adjusted summery of all causes mortality is:
- A. Multivariate analysis
- B. Proportional mortality rate
- C. Regression analysis
- D. Life table

73. Best comparison of health status of two populations is done by:
- A. CDR
- B. Proportional mortality rate
- C. Standardized mortality rate
- D. Specific death rate

74. The burden of disease is best represented by:
- A. DALY's
- B. PQLI
- C. Case fatality rate
- D. IMR

75. Death rates of two countries are compared by:
- A. Proportional death rate
- B. ASDR
- C. Standardized mortality rate
- D. CDR

76. Among the following the best indicator of health in a community is:
- A. MMR
- B. Life expectancy
- C. IMR
- D. NMR

77. Most useful single measure of mortality is:
- A. CDR
- B. ASDR
- C. Proportional mortality rate
- D. Case fatality rate

---

71 A 72 D 73 C 74 A 75 C 76 C
77 B

78. In international death certificate, most important information to entered is:
- **A.** Disease directly related to death
- **B.** Underlying cause of death
- **C.** Age at death
- **D.** Significant associated condition that attributed to death

79. About direct standardization all are true *except:*
- **A.** ASDRs are not needed
- **B.** A standard population is needed
- **C.** Two populations are compared
- **D.** Populations should be comparable

80. Denominator in CDR is:
- **A.** Total number of births
- **B.** Population at risk
- **C.** Mid year population
- **D.** None of the above

81. Which of the following factors influence CDR?
- **A.** Age
- **B.** Sex
- **C.** Marital status
- **D.** All of the above

82. Standardize mortality ratio is:
- **A.** $\frac{\text{Observed deaths}}{\text{Expected deaths}} \times \text{Standard factor}$
- **B.** $\frac{\text{Observed deaths}}{\text{Expected deaths}} \times 100$
- **C.** $\frac{\text{Observed deaths} + \text{Expected deaths}}{2}$
- **D.** $\frac{\text{Observed deaths} - \text{Expected deahs}}{\text{Expected deaths}}$

78 B **79 A** **80 C** **81 D** **82 B**

83. The number of deaths in people about 60 year as a percentage of total deaths of all ages is known as:

A. CDR
B. Expectancy of life
C. Proportional mortality rate
D. ASDR

84. All are true statements about proportional mortality rate *except:*

A. It is computed for communicable disease as a hole
B. It depends upon two variables
C. Proportional mortality rate does not indicates the risk of dying from the disease
D. It is used only when the total population is known

85. Proportional mortality rate is defined as:

A. $\dfrac{\text{Number of deaths due to disease in a year}}{\text{Total number of diseased persons}} \times 100$

B. $\dfrac{\text{Number of deaths due to disease in a year}}{\text{Total deaths from all causes during that year}} \times 100$

C. $\dfrac{\text{Number of deaths due to disease in a year}}{\text{Population at risk}} \times 100$

D. $\dfrac{\text{Number of deaths due to disease in a year}}{\text{Mid year population}} \times 1000$

83 C 84 D 85 B

86. All of the following are true for MMR, *except:*
- **A.** It requires the number of live births
- **B.** It requires an assessment of cause of death
- **C.** It depends on deaths of women at any age
- **D.** It is based on deaths of women within 6 weeks of delivery

87. All are true about standardized mortality ratio *except:*
- **A.** Total number of deaths per year
- **B.** It is useful for comparison of two populations
- **C.** Ratio of observed deaths and expected deaths
- **D.** Can be calculated even if age specific death is not available

88. The National Population Policy 2000 aims to achieve NRR = 1 by the year:
- **A.** 2005 **B.** 2010
- **C.** 2015 **D.** 2020

89. In 2001 census, the percentage of people belonging to age 60 years and above is:
- **A.** 2% **B.** 4%
- **C.** 7% **D.** 10%

90. If TFR in a population is 5 per women, the GRR is:
- **A.** 2.5 **B.** 5
- **C.** 10 **D.** None of the above

91. Nuclear family consists of:
- **A.** Husband and wife only
- **B.** Husband, wife and son
- **C.** Husband, wife and dependent children
- **D.** Husband, wife, father, mother and children

92. All of the following factors are considered in Human Development Index *except:*
- **A.** Income **B.** Life expectancy
- **C.** Literacy **D.** IMR

---

86 C 87 A 88 B 89 C 90 A 91 C 92 D

Biostatistics

ten

Health Information, Education and Planning

1. All of the following are required for health Information system, *except:*
   A. System should be population based
   B. System should be problem oriented
   C. System should express information briefly
   D. System should not be periodically reviewed

2. Which of the following is not related to health information system?
   A. Demography
   B. Environmental health statistics
   C. Notification of diseases
   D. Geography

3. Information regarding disabled persons in the country is not available from:
   A. Census 2001
   B. National Sample Survey 1991
   C. SRS 1998
   D. None of the above

4. Cause of death can not be obtained by:
   A. Medical certificate of death
   B. Census report
   C. Verbal autopsy
   D. Postmortem examination

1 D 2 D 3 C 4 B

5. **Lay reporting involves collection of information by:**
   - **A.** Non-professional health workers
   - **B.** Village health guide
   - **C.** Medical Officers
   - **D.** ANMs

6. **All of the following are true about notification of diseases, *except:***
   - **A.** Primary purpose is to effect prevention and control of the disease
   - **B.** Covers a large part of the total sickness in the community
   - **C.** Provides information about fluctuations in disease frequency
   - **D.** Provides early warning about outbreaks of disease frequency

7. **The Rehabilitation Council of India Act has been enacted on:**
   - **A.** 15th July 1990
   - **B.** 7th August 1992
   - **C.** 31st July 1993
   - **D.** 15th March 2000

8. **All of the following factors related to referral system, *except:***
   - **A.** How to attract and retain clients
   - **B.** How the client will go to the referral point
   - **C.** To whom the client should contact at referral site
   - **D.** What documentation should be given to client at the referral site

9. **Hardly–Weinberg law is related to:**
   - **A.** Health economics
   - **B.** Social medicine
   - **C.** Population genetics
   - **D.** Population control strategies

10. **The SAFE strategy has been developed for the control of:**
    - **A.** Refractive error
    - **B.** Diabetes mellitus
    - **C.** Onchocerciasis
    - **D.** Trachoma

---

5 A 6 B 7 C 8 A 9 C 10 D

11. **Double edged sword is:**
    A. Chlorine
    B. Lead
    C. Selenium
    D. Fluorine

12. **Family Welfare Programme's goal is reach CPR of:**
    A. 20%
    B. 40%
    C. 60%
    D. 100%

13. **In India, Rabies free zone is:**
    A. Goa
    B. Lakshadeep
    C. Nagaland
    D. Sikkim

14. **Pulse Polio Immunization Programme was launched on:**
    A. 6th December 1994
    B. 14th November 1995
    C. 9th December 1995
    D. 7th December 1996

15. **Under Integrated Rural Development Programme all are provided *except:***
    A. Employment
    B. Bank loans
    C. Resources
    D. Subsidies

16. **Family Planning Association of India has its Headquarter in:**
    A. New Delhi
    B. Kolkata
    C. Mumbai
    D. Chennai

17. **The programme in which CARE has provided maximum help in India is:**
    A. Immunization
    B. Mid-day meal scheme
    C. Family planning
    D. Provision of medical equipments

18. **ESI act provides for:**
    A. Medical benefit
    B. Sickness benefit
    C. Maternity benefit
    D. All of the above

---

11 D 12 C 13 B 14 C 15 A 16 C
17 B 18 D

19. Society is defined as:

A. System of social relationship between individuals

B. Social relationship between families

C. Intervention of individuals and families

D. Relationship of individual, family and the country

20. Small for date babies are prevented by:

A. Spacing in births

B. Antenatal care

C. Nutritional supplement

D. Immunization

21. Living standard of people is best assessed by:

A. IMR

B. MMR

C. Death rate

D. PQLI

22. Positive health indicators of nutritional status include all of the following, *except:*

A. Heightof school children at school entry

B. Prevalence of LBW

C. Anthropometric measurements of pre school children

D. Weight of pregnant mothers

23. Main draw back of calculating incidence of disease using hospital records is:

A. Poor maintenance of records

B. Sub clinical cases not admitted

C. Denominator not well defined

D. None of the above

24. The most common industrial disease of the employees is:

A. Chronic bronchitis

B. Occupational dermatosis

C. Emphysema

D. Silicosis

---

19 A 20 A 21 C 22 D 23 C 24 A

25. In a society a social act which is considered natural and right is referred to as:
 A. Taboo
 B. Custom
 C. Ritual
 D. Tradition

26. Retrospective study of case sheets and evaluation of medical data is called:
 A. Medical evaluation
 B. Medical audit
 C. Performance evaluation
 D. Professional screening

27. TRIAGE means:
 A. Catering to patients with major injuries first
 B. Dividing patients into categories based on necessities for action and resources available
 C. Seeing only emergency cases
 D. Seeing all patients as they come into the casualty adhoc basis

28. Behavioral sciences are all *except:*
 A. Psychology
 B. Sociology
 C. Anthropology
 D. Political science

29. Optimal healthy life includes all of the following *except:*
 A. Moderate physical exercise
 B. Sufficient nutrition
 C. Regular swimming
 D. Blood and urine examination at least twice a year

30. Which of the following is not true about Didactic method of communication?
 A. Learning is authoritative
 B. Knowledge is imposed
 C. To influence human behavior
 D. No feedback from audience

25 B **26 B** **27 B** **28 D** **29 C** **30 B**

31. To increase awareness of rural population towards small family norms, the best method is:

A. Radio
B. Television
C. Posters and charts exhibition
D. Role playing

32. Most common channel of communication is:

A. Face to face interaction
B. Folk dances
C. Film show
D. Dramas

33. Which of the following is not a Two-way communication:

A. Group discussion B. Symposium
C. Seminars D. Lectures

34. All of the following are the barriers to communication, *except:*

A. Illiteracy
B. Socio economic status
C. Attitudes
D. Level of intelligence

35. All are true about mass communication, *except:*

A. Suits local needs
B. Rapid
C. Undistorted information
D. Cost effective

36. The entire communication process related to a health issue basically intends to change:

A. Awareness level
B. Behavior
C. Attitudes and practices
D. Sensitivity and receptivity thresholds

37. Which of the following is a Socratic method of teaching?

A. Exhibition B. Lecture
C. Audio video aids D. Panel discussion

---

31 D 32 A 33 D 34 B 35 A 36 A
37 D

38. All of the following statements are true for group discussion, *except:*
- **A.** Each member should prepare a topic to discuss
- **B.** It is two-way communication
- **C.** An effective group is composed of 6-12 persons
- **D.** The team leader initiates and guides the discussion

39. All of the following features are related to mass media education, *except:*
- **A.** Rapid and controlled
- **B.** Easy understanding
- **C.** Interesting and widely approachable
- **D.** Deals with local problems of community

40. All are features of health education, *except:*
- **A.** Develops reflexive behavior
- **B.** Disciplines primitive desires
- **C.** Appeals to reason
- **D.** Knowledge is actively required

41. Health education is:
- **A.** To prevent the disease
- **B.** Health promotion
- **C.** Health distortion
- **D.** To educate school children

42. Health education aims at:
- **A.** Appealing to emotions
- **B.** Acquiring knowledge through self-reliant activity
- **C.** Spoon feeding of knowledge
- **D.** Installing knowledge in the minds of the people

43. Following are used in planning of health education, *except:*
- **A.** Catchy slogans
- **B.** Using simple words
- **C.** Ensuring community participation
- **D.** Considering the felt needs

38 A 39 D 40 A 41 B 42 B 43 A

44. The objective of health education is to:
- **A.** Teach personal hygiene to community
- **B.** Teach school children preventive medicine
- **C.** Effect chance in health practices of people and in their knowledge and attitudes towards the health
- **D.** Make the people aware about disease prevention and health promotion

45. Non-formal education is a component of:
- **A.** School health programme
- **B.** ICDS scheme
- **C.** ESI scheme
- **D.** None of the above

46. Which of the following is a very effective method of health education to bring out change in health behavior of people?
- **A.** Panel discussion
- **B.** Group discussion
- **C.** Workshops and seminars
- **D.** Film show

47. Which of the following is true about Symposium?
- **A.** Series of speech are presented on a selected topic
- **B.** Two-way communication
- **C.** Demonstration is carried out for the topic
- **D.** There is a discussion among members on the subject

48. The best teaching opportunity for a female health worker in community is while:
- **A.** Demonstrating to a group of mother
- **B.** Examining mothers and children
- **C.** Completing the records
- **D.** None of the above

44 C 45 B 46 B 47 D 48 A

49. Which of the following method is useful educational method for school children?

A. Demonstration
B. Group discussion
C. Role playing
D. Simulation exercise

50. Which is the most potent media for general public education?

A. News papers
B. Magazines
C. Radio
D. TV

51. The best method of teaching in urban–slum about ORS is:

A. Flash cards
B. Role play
C. Film show
D. Demonstration

52. Which of the following is not a correct principle of health?

A. Unknown to known
B. Reinforcement
C. Participation
D. Soil, seed and sower

53. Which of the following is not true about lecture as health education method?

A. Giving basic information
B. One way of communication
C. Large number of points are covered in a short time
D. Group should not be more than 30

54. WHO constitution was made in:

A. 1947
B. 1952
C. 1957
D. 1960

55. Primary health care is a concept by:

A. UNICEF and accepted by all countries
B. Common Wealth countries and accepted by all countries
C. WHO and accepted by India
D. India and accepted by all countries

---

49 C **50 D** **51 D** **52 A** **53 C** **54 A**
55 C

56. ANM does not work of:

A. Birth death statistics
B. Immunization
C. Distribution of condoms
D. Malaria surveillance

57. Sub centre in a hilly area caters to population of:

A. 1000 **B.** 2000
C. 3000 **D.** 5000

58. Anganwadi workers are under the administration of:

A. Primary Health Centre
B. Ministry of Health and Family Welfare
C. Ministry of Labour
D. ICDS

59. Health guide (male) is at level of:

A. Sub-centre
B. PHC
C. CHC
D. Village

60. In hilly area, PHC controls to population of:

A. 10,000 **B.** 20,000
C. 30,000 **D.** 40,000

61. A Community Health Centre:

A. Is controlled by the Panchayat
B. Has specialists on Ophthalmologist and Orthopedics
C. Covers a population of 1.20 lacs
D. Is governed by District Magistrate

62. PHC can be differentiated from dispensary by:

A. Located in rural area
B. Headed by Medical Officer
C. Provides essential care
D. Provides integrated health services

---

56 D 57 C 58 D 59 D 60 B 61 C
62 D

63. Bed turn over rate in a hospital is:
A. Number of beds, discharged in a day
B. Number of beds, vacant in a particular day
C. Number of beds, occupied in a particular day
D. Number of beds required

64. The UNICEF was established in:
A. 1929
B. 1946
C. 1952
D. 1960

65. WHO day is on:
A. 7th April
B. 21st May
C. 2nd August
D. 31st December

66. A type-II urban family welfare centre caters to populations of:
A. 5000-10,000
B. 25,000-50,000
C. 50,000-80,000
D. 1,00,000 and above

67. Which one of the following strategies is aimed at AIDS control in India?
A. Detection and Isolation of HIV infected persons in the community
B. Immunoprophylaxis of the risk groups
C. Community education towards behavioral change
D. Detection and treatment of AIDS cases in the community

68. Which one of the following dimension is not addressed during a social research survey?
A. Social Structure
B. Social Institutions
C. Social Pathology
D. Social Psychology

69. Community health worker will learn best by taking part in:
A. Demonstration
B. Group discussion
C. Seminars
D. Workshops

63 A 64 B 65 A 66 B 67 C 68 B
69 B

70. A technique adopted by health management in which a critical review and evaluation of programme is made and represented in the form of a diagram is termed as:

A. Information system
B. Information, education and communication
C. System analysis
D. PERT

71. The assessment of a health programme where the benefit is expressed in terms of results achieved is called:

A. Cost containment
B. Cost benefit analysis
C. Cost accounting
D. Cost effectiveness analysis

72. A network is graphic plan of all events and activities to be completed in order to reach an objective. Which one of the following is a common type of network analysis?

A. Input–output analysis
B. Critical path method
C. Planning, programming and budgeting system
D. System analysis

73. In solving public health problems, long lasting solutions can be obtained from:

A. Participatory approach
B. Educational approach
C. Regulatory approach
D. Service approach

74. In the critical path method of network analysis, the critical path is the:

A. Shortest
B. Longest
C. Cheapest
D. Costliest

---

70 D **71 D** **72 B** **73 C** **74 B**

75. Administrative failure in malaria control included all of the following, *except:*

A. Resistance of the parasites to chloroquine
B. Shortage of inacticides
C. Deficiency in recruiting labour for spray work
D. Shortage of anti-malarial drugs

76. To match the limited resources to accomplish a definite objective by eliminating wasteful expenditure in the shortest possible time, is the definition of:

A. Management
B. Planning
C. Organization
D. Evaluation

77. Feasibility of a program is defined by:

A. Number of staff
B. Competency
C. Financial backup
D. Dedication of workers

78. The project management technique used for time scheduling and monitoring is:

A. Network analysis
B. Budgeting
C. Accounting and auditing
D. Cost benefit analysis

79 Time taken for any project is estimated by:

A. Work sampling
B. Network analysis
C. System analysis
D. Input-output analysis

80. Panchayat Raj means:

A. Primary health care
B. Rural Health Development
C. Local self rule government
D. Rural leadership

75 A 76 B 77 C 78 A 79 B 80 C

81. Primary health care includes all of the following, *except:*

A. Family planning services
B. MCH and immunization services
C. Health education regarding water disinfection
D. Specialized health services

82. All of the following are related to primary health care, *except:*

A. Services rendered by medical officers
B. Community participation
C. Appropriate technology
D. Inter-Sectorial coordination

83. PERT is a management technique for:

A. Input-output analysis
B. System analysis
C. Cost effectiveness analysis
D. Network analysis

84. PERT is based on:

A. Qualitative methods
B. Quantitative methods
C. Behavioral sciences
D. None of the above

85. Which of the following is not related to SWOT analysis?

A. The process analyzing weaknesses of programme
B. To analyze strengths and opportunities that exist outside the programme
C. Auditing the programme time to time
D. To understand threats that exist in and out of the programme

86. Social marketing is related to:

A. Health Products
B. Health Services
C. Health Education
D. All of the above

---

81 D 82 A 83 D 84 A 85 C 86 D

87. Which of the following is not applied to social marketing?

A. Marketing to condoms and Mala-D Tablets
B. Immunization
C. Counseling for drug de-addiction
D. Surveillance of disease

88. NACO has been setup in:

A. 1981 B. 1990
C. 1992 D. 1995

89. GOBIFFF campaign has been popularized by:

A. WHO B. UNICEF
C. CARE D. World Bank

90. National Rural Health Mission has been launched in:

A. 1996 B. 2000
C. 2001 D. 2005

87 D 88 C 89 B 90 D

Part-II
Epidemiology

eleven

Concepts of Epidemiology

1. **Epidemiology involves study of:**
   - A. Disease frequency
   - B. Distribution of disease
   - C. Determinants of disease
   - D. All of the above
2. **Epidemiologic studies of disease usually involve:**
   - A. Discarding the clinical knowledge of disease
   - B. Both people with and without the disease under study
   - C. Relating local cases to the national population
   - D. Emphasizing the cases of advanced disease
3. **Which of the following epidemiological studies deals with risk factors of disease?**
   - A. Analytical Epidemiology
   - B. Descriptive Epidemiology
   - C. Experimental Epidemiology
   - D. None of the above
4. **The basic goal of epidemiological research is to:**
   - A. Eliminate all bias
   - B. Reject the Null hypothesis
   - C. Maximize external validity
   - D. Compare two groups that differ by exposure or outcome

---

1 D 2 B 3 A 4 D

5. **Which of the following is true about making comparison in epidemiological approach?**
   A. The comparability can be ensured by randomization
   B. Both the study and control groups should be similar
   C. Random allocation is not possible in case of control and cohort study
   D. All of the above

6. **Epidemiology deals the study of:**
   A. Epidemic diseases
   B. Communicable diseases
   C. Risk factors of diseases
   D. All health related events and states in a population

7. **Experimental epidemiology deals with:**
   A. Epidemics
   B. Screening of disease
   C. Intervention
   D. Early diagnosis

8. **Study of time, place and person is called as:**
   A. Descriptive epidemiology
   B. Experimental epidemiology
   C. Analytical epidemiology
   D. Randomized controlled trial

9. **Epidemiological triad is:**
   A. Agent, Host and Environment
   B. Agent, Host and Vector
   C. Carrier, Environment and Vector
   D. Agent, Treatment and Reservoir

10. **Epidemiological triad includes all the following *except:***
   A. Agent
   B. Environment
   C. Reservoir
   D. Host

---

5 D 6 D 7 C 8 A 9 A 10 C

11. Course of disease process without any intervention is:

A. Natural history of disease
B. Epidemiological triad
C. Epidemiology
D. Disability

12. In which of the following epidemiological measurements is numerator not a component of denominator?

A. Percentage
B. Proportion
C. Rate
D. Ratio

13. The study of inter-relationship of all the living things is called:

A. Ecology
B. Epidemiology
C. Anthropology
D. Social pathology

11 A 12 D 13 A

twelve

Measurements in Epidemiology

1. The basic requirements of epidemiological measurements include all *except:*

A. Applicability
B. Reliability
C. Accuracy
D. Validity

2. The first step for conducting an epidemiologic investigation is to:

A. Determine the case count
B. Determine the population at risk
C. Calculate the incubation period
D. Verify the diagnosis

3. Which of the following expresses a relation in size between two random quantities?

A. Rate
B. Ratio
C. Proportion
D. Percentage

4. A rate in disease measurement is a statement of:

A. The risk of developing a condition
B. The force of infection
C. The speed at which a communicable disease spreads
D. The speed at which a non-communicable disease spreads

1 A 2 D 3 B 4 A

5. Incidence is defined as:

A. Number of new cases occurring during a specified period in given population

B. Number of old cases present during a specified period in given population

C. Number of cases occurring in a given population

D. Number of cases existing in a given population at a given time

6. The risk of acquiring a disease is measured by:

A. Incidence rate

B. Prevalence rate

C. Incidence rate times the average duration of the disease

D. Prevalence rate times the average duration of the disease

7. Incidence rate is measured by:

A. Case control study

B. Cohort study

C. Cross-sectional study

D. Intervention study

8. All the following include the uses of incidence rate *except:*

A. It reflects the change in etiology of disease

B. It reflects the prognostic factors

C. It indicates failure or ineffectiveness of the current control programme

D. It suggests the need for new disease control or preventive programme

9. In a community an increase in new cases denotes:

A. Increase in incidence rate

B. Increase in prevalence rate

C. Decrease in incidence rate

D. Decrease in prevalence rate

---

5 A 6 A 7 B 8 B 9 A

10. Incidence is calculated by:

A. Retrospective study
B. Prospective study
C. Cross sectional study
D. Random study

11. The following are morbidity indicators, *except:*

A. Incidence rate
B. Duration of stay in hospital
C. Notification rates
D. Life expectancy

12. If incidence of disease is 100 per year and duration of disease is 2 years in a population of 5000. What is prevalence?

A. 10 per 1000 B. 20 per 1000
C. 40 per 1000 D. 80 per 1000

13. Prevalence of a disease affects:

A. Predictive value B. Relative risk
C. Sensitivity D. Specificity

14. Prevalence of TB infection in a community is indicated by:

A. The proportion of individuals with a positive reaction to the standard tuberculin test
B. The percentage of new cases in a year
C. The proportion of the population whose sputum is positive for the tubercle bacillus
D. The number of individuals who have radiographic evidence

15. The most sensitive index to assess the transmission of leprosy under NLEP is:

A. Incidence rate B. Detection rate
C. Coverage rate D. Disability rate

16. In calculating incidence of AIDS, the denominator is:

A. Total population
B. Population at risk
C. Mid year population
D. Observed population

---

10 B 11 C 12 C 13 A 14 A 15 A
16 B

17. Prevalence is useful:
- **A.** To identify potential high risk population
- **B.** For the efficacy of preventive and curative measure
- **C.** To control disease
- **D.** For distribution of disease

18. Total number of cases at a given point of time in a given population is:
- **A.** Prevalence rate
- **B.** Attack rate
- **C.** Epidemic
- **D.** Incidence rate

19. When a new treatment is developed that prevents death but does not produce recovery from a disease, the following will occur:
- **A.** Incidence of the disease will increase
- **B.** Incidence of the disease will decrease
- **C.** Prevalence of the disease will decrease
- **D.** Prevalence of the disease will increase

20. A disease has 3 times more incidence in females as compared to males with same prevalence in both males and females. True statement is:
- **A.** Less fatality in males
- **B.** Increase fatality in females
- **C.** More survival in females
- **D.** Better prognosis in males

21. In trachoma survey of a community the incidence of inflammatory trachoma was 2% and incidence of cicartricial trachoma was 3%. Which of the following statements is true:
- **A.** Problem is still there in the community
- **B.** Problem was prevalent in past but now under control
- **C.** Problem was not prevalent but now prevalent
- **D.** Problem was prevalent in past and still prevalent

---

17 A 18 A 19 D 20 B 21 B

22. **In a stable situation:**
   A. Prevalence = Incidence + duration of disease
   B. Incidence = Prevalence + duration of disease
   C. Incidence = Prevalence × duration of disease
   D. Prevalence = Incidence × duration of disease

23. **All of the following statements regarding the prevalence are true, *except:***
   A. It is a rate
   B. It is a ratio
   C. Duration of disease effects prevalence
   D. Numerator and denominator are separate entities

24. **If I, indicates incidence; P, indicates prevalence, and D, denotes duration of diseases, then the relationship between prevalence and incidence is expressed as:**
   A. P = I ÷ D
   B. I = P × D
   C. P = I × D
   D. I = 1 – P/D

25. **Prevalence of a disease affects:**
   A. Predictive value
   B. Specificity
   C. Relative risk
   D. Sensitivity

26. **A particularly useful measure of events that can occur repeatedly in individual subjects under observation is:**
   A. Incidence rate
   B. Period prevalence
   C. Risk
   D. Incidence density

27. **All are true about attack rate *except:***
   A. It is expressed as percentage
   B. It is a type of prevalence rate
   C. It reflects extent of epidemic
   D. It is used when population is exposed to risk for a limited period of time

---

22 D 23 A 24 C 25 A 26 D 27 B

28. There are 120 children in a community, out of whom 32 were immunized against measles; 3 of them acquire measles simultaneously; subsequently 17 get measles. Assuming the efficacy of the vaccine to be 100%. What is the secondary attack rate?

A. 20%   B. 25%
C. 27%   D. 5%

29. Secondary attack rate is calculated from:

A. Maximum incubation period
B. Minimum incubation period
C. Average incubation period
D. None of the above

30. Secondary attack rate reflects:

A. Fatality of disease
B. Communicability of disease
C. Infectivity of disease
D. Severity of disease

31. An important measure of the communicability of a disease is:

A. Case fatality rate
B. Infection rate
C. Secondary attack rate
D. None of the above

32. The formula used for calculating secondary attack rate is:

A. $\dfrac{\text{No. of contacts developing disease in one maximum incubation period}}{\text{Total number of susceptible contacts}} \times 100$

B. $\dfrac{\text{No. of contacts developing disease in one minimum incubation period}}{\text{Total number of susceptible contacts}} \times 100$

C. $\dfrac{\text{Number of persons developing disease}}{\text{Total number of persons exposed}} \times 100$

D. None of the above

28 A   29 A   30 B   31 C   32 A

33. Which of the following is reflected by secondary attack rate?

A. Fatality B. Severity
C. Communicability D. Susceptibility

34. Secondary attack is useful to determine:

A. Attack rate in vaccinated and unvaccinated population
B. Whether a disease of unknown etiology is communicable or not
C. Evaluation of effectiveness and control measures
D. All of the above

35. Denominator in secondary attack rate is:

A. Number of contacts developing disease
B. Number of contacts developing disease within maximum incubation period
C. Total number of persons developing disease
D. Total number of susceptible exposed

36. Denominator in Crude death rate is:

A. Total number of births
B. Population at risk
C. Mid year population
D. None of the above

37. Which of the following factors influences CDR?

A. Age B. Sex
C. Marital status D. All of the above

38. All are true statements about proportional mortality rate *except:*

A. It is computed for communicable disease as a whole
B. It depends upon two variables
C. Proportional mortality rate does not indicate the risk of dying from the disease
D. It is used only when the total population is known

---

33 C 34 D 35 D 36 C 37 D 38 D

39. Proportional mortality rate is:

A. $\frac{\text{No. of deaths due to disease in a year}}{\text{Total No. of diseased persons}} \times 100$

B. $\frac{\text{No. of deaths due to disease in a year}}{\text{Total deaths from all causes during that year}} \times 100$

C. $\frac{\text{No. of deaths due to disease in a year}}{\text{Population at risk}} \times 100$

D. $\frac{\text{No. of deaths due to disease in a year}}{\text{Mid year population}} \times 100$

40. The number of deaths in people above 60 years as a percentage of total deaths of all ages is known as:

A. Crude death rate
B. Expectancy of life
C. Proportional mortality rate
D. Age specific death rate

41. Most useful single measure of mortality is:

A. Crude death rate
B. Age-specific death rate
C. Proportional mortality rate
D. Case fatality rate

42. In International death certificate, most important information to be entered is:

A. Disease directly related to death
B. Underlying cause of death
C. Age at death
D. Significant associated condition that contributed to death

43. An indicator of severity of disease is:

A. Case fatality rate
B. Incidence rate
C. Prevalence rate
D. Cause specific death rate

---

39 B 40 C 41 B 42 B 43 A

44. Standardized mortality ratio is:

A. $\frac{\text{Observed deaths} \times \text{Standard factor}}{\text{Expected deaths}}$

B. $\frac{\text{Observed deaths}}{\text{Expected deaths}} \times 100$

C. $\frac{\text{Observed deaths} + \text{Expected deaths}}{2}$

D. $\frac{\text{Observed deaths} - \text{Expected deaths}}{\text{Expected deaths}}$

45. All are true about community diagnosis *except:*

A. Age-specific death rate
B. Age-sex pyramid
C. Vital statistics
D. Incidence rate

46. Case fatality rate indicates:

A. Severity of disease
B. Incidence
C. Prevalence
D. Morbidity of disease

47. Case fatality rate is:

A. Percentage **B.** Proportion
C. Ratio **D.** Constant

48. Case fatality rate for a given disease refers to:

A. A fatal outcome of any disease
B. Percentage of deaths among cases of the disease
C. Cause specific mortality rate due to the disease
D. Proportion of deaths due to the disease among all deaths from all cases

49. The Case fatality rate measures:

A. Pathogenecity **B.** Infectivity
C. Mortality **D.** Virulence

44 B 45 A 46 A 47 C 48 B 49 D

50. During a six months period, 10 cases of Hanta virus pulmonary syndrome are reported in a hospital, and out of them 3 cases died. Which of the following rate/ratio would be 33.3 percentage?

A. The attack rate
B. The crude death rate
C. The standardized mortality ratio
D. The case fatality ratio

51. Which of the following indicates the severity of illness in a given population?

A. Incidence rate
B. Prevalence
C. Proportional mortality rate
D. Case fatality rate

52. In an epidemiological study, the incidence of disease in female is more than in male but the prevalence is equal in both. What does it indicate?

A. Female harbours disease for long duration
B. Disease is of less duration in male
C. Case fatality is more in female
D. Mortality in male is more

53. A useful index to measure the lethality of an acute infectious disease is:

A. Incidence rate
B. Attack rate
C. Case fatality rate
D. None of the above

54. Which is not true about case fatality rate?

A. Case fatality rate varies in different epidemics
B. It is the ratio of deaths to cases
C. It is closely related to virulence
D. The time interval is specified

---

50 D **51 D** **52 C** **53 C** **54 D**

55. The killing power of a disease is represented by:

A. Attack rate
B. Case fatality ratio
C. Proportional mortality
D. Crude death rate

56. In an outbreak of a disease in a village of 3500 population, 40 cases have occurred and 8 have died. Case fatality rate is:

A. 0.2% **B.** 20%
C. 8% **D.** None of the above

57. Pathogenecity is calculated by:

A. $\dfrac{\text{Number of deaths}}{\text{Number of persons with disease}}$

B. $\dfrac{\text{Number with disease}}{\text{Number infected}}$

C. $\dfrac{\text{Number infected}}{\text{Number exposed}}$

D. $\dfrac{\text{Number with serious condition}}{\text{Number with disease}}$

58. Which of the following is true for assessment of incidence of a disease in community?

A. It requires a retrospective study
B. It requires a cross-sectional study
C. It requires a prospective study
D. None of the above

55 B 56 B 57 B 58 C

Epidemiology

thirteen

Epidemiologic Methods

Descriptive Epidemiology

1. Which of the following is an advantage of a retrospective study?

A. It may be used to study etiology of a rare disease
B. There is little or no bias in assessment of exposure to the factor
C. It is possible to determine the true incidence rate of the disease
D. Dependence on recall by subjects in the study is minimized

2. A major weakness of retrospective studies of the role of a suspected factor in the etiology of a disease as compared with prospective studies is that:

A. They are more costly and take longer time
B. There may be bias in determining the presence or absence of the suspected factor
C. It is more difficult to obtain controls
D. There may be bias in determining the presence or absence of the resulting disease

1 A   2 B

3. A retrospective study is characterized by all except the following:
- **A.** Incidence rate may be computed
- **B.** It is relatively inexpensive
- **C.** Assessment of past exposure may be biased
- **D.** One selects controls without the disease

4. Which of the following study is also called retrospective study:
- **A.** Cross sectional study
- **B.** Case control study
- **C.** Experimental study
- **D.** None of the above

5. A retrospective study is characterized by all *except:*
- **A.** It is relatively inexpensive
- **B.** Incidence rates may be computed
- **C.** Relative risk may be estimated from the results
- **D.** One selects controls without the disease

6. All the following can be obtained from prospective study *except:*
- **A.** Incidence rate
- **B.** Prevalence rate
- **C.** Relative risk
- **D.** Attributable risk

7. In a prospective study of a disease the cohort originally selected consisted of:
- **A.** Subjects without the disease
- **B.** Subjects with the factor under investigation
- **C.** Subjects without the factor under investigation
- **D.** Subjects who are found to have the disease

8. All of the following are true about cross-sectional study, *except:*
- **A.** Tells about duration of disease
- **B.** Tells about distribution of disease
- **C.** Does not provide information about incidence
- **D.** Based on single observation at one point of time

---

3 A   4 B   5 B   6 B   7 A   8 A

9. Which of the following epidemiological methods uses individuals as unit study:

- **A.** Case control study
- **B.** Cross sectional study
- **C.** Randomized controlled trials
- **D.** All of the above

10. Which of the following study is also known as prevalence study:

- **A.** Cross sectional study
- **B.** Cohort study
- **C.** Case control study
- **D.** Longitudinal study

11. A study conducted on infant mortality during the period of January 2003 to December 2003, it would be:

- **A.** Cohort study
- **B.** Retrospective study
- **C.** Prospective study
- **D.** None of the above

12. In which of the following study there is an active attempt to change a disease determinant or the progress of a disease:

- **A.** Experimental study
- **B.** Observational study
- **C.** Analytical study
- **D.** None of the above

13. False about longitudinal study is:

- **A.** To study natural history of disease
- **B.** Very economic
- **C.** Incidence can not be measured
- **D.** Identifies risk factor

14. Which of the following statements is not true about cross sectional studies:

- **A.** Help in identifying risk factors of disease
- **B.** Provides information regarding natural history of disease
- **C.** More useful for chronic disease
- **D.** None of the above

9 D 10 A 11 B 12 A 13 C 14 A

15. Which of the following study is best for calculating the incidence of a disease:

- **A.** Case control study
- **B.** Cohort study
- **C.** Cross sectional study
- **D.** Longitudinal study

16. Prevalence of disease is estimated from:

- **A.** Double blind study
- **B.** Case control study
- **C.** Cohort study
- **D.** Cross sectional study

17. Host factor strongly related to disease is:

- **A.** Sex
- **B.** Marital status
- **C.** Age
- **D.** Occupation

18. Community intervention studies are:

- **A.** Cross sectional studies
- **B.** Case control studies
- **C.** Cohort studies
- **D.** Field trials

19. Epidemic refers to:

- **A.** An attack rate in excess of 10 per 1000 population
- **B.** A disease that has a low rate of occurrence but that is constantly present in a community
- **C.** The occurrence of illnesses of similar nature clearly in excess of the normal expectation for that population at that time
- **D.** Diseases of the respiratory system that occur seasonally

20. All are features of point source epidemic *except:*

- **A.** Epidemic tends to be explosive
- **B.** Epidemic continuous over more than one incubation period
- **C.** Epidemic curve fluctuates very rapidly
- **D.** Epidemic curve shows no secondary waves

15 D   16 D   17 C   18 D   19 C   20 B

21. Bhopal gas tragedy is an example of:
- **A.** Slow epidemic
- **B.** Point source epidemic
- **C.** Propagated epidemic
- **D.** None of the above

22. Epidemic occurring every three years is called:
- **A.** Cyclic trend
- **B.** Annular disease
- **C.** Secular trend
- **D.** Pandemic

23. Progressive increase or decrease in occurrence of a disease or along period of time is known as:
- **A.** Seasonal trend
- **B.** Secular trend
- **C.** Cyclic trend
- **D.** Exotic trend

24. Secular trend refers to:
- **A.** Change of pattern over a long period of time
- **B.** Decrease in prevalence of disease
- **C.** Gradual change in a particular direction
- **D.** Occurs due to naturally occurring variation in herd immunity

25. Secular tend of disease refers to its:
- **A.** Current status
- **B.** Seasonal trend
- **C.** Occurrence due to variation in herd immunity
- **D.** Change of pattern over a long period of time

26. Serial interval is:
- **A.** Time gap between index case and primary case
- **B.** Time gap between primary and secondary case
- **C.** Time taken for a person from infection to develop maximum infectivity
- **D.** The time taken from infection till a person infects another person

---

21 B **22 A** **23 B** **24 A** **25 D** **26 B**

27. All are true regarding Point source epidemic *except:*

A. Children are most commonly affected
B. All cases occur abruptly and simultaneously
C. Occurs within a specified period
D. No secondary waves

28. False regarding a propagated epidemic is:

A. No secondary waves
B. Spread depends on herd immunity
C. Person to person transmission occurs
D. Slow rise

29. All of the following features are true about cross – sectional study *except:*

A. All cases are seen at one point of time
B. Cause and effect relationship can be established
C. Follow up is not a necessary feature
D. More useful for chronic disease

30. All are true for propagated epidemic curve *except:*

A. Many peaks
B. Steep and abrupt onset
C. More than one incubation period
D. Prolonged epidemic tail

31. Food poisoning is an example of:

A. Point source epidemic
B. Propagated epidemic
C. Continuous epidemic
D. Modern epidemic

32. Seasonal variation of a disease can be assessed by:

A. Using mortality rates
B. Using survival rates
C. Comparing incidence of disease
D. Comparing prevalence of disease

---

27 A 28 A 29 B 30 B 31 A 32 C

33. Cyclic trend is seen in all *except:*
- **A.** Chicken Pox
- **B.** Measles
- **C.** Influenza
- **D.** None of the above

34. All of the following show seasonal trend *except:*
- **A.** Measles
- **B.** Sun stroke
- **C.** Automobile accidents
- **D.** Cholera

35. When a disease frequency is measured over a period of several years of decades, it is called:
- **A.** Secular trend
- **B.** Seasonal trend
- **C.** Cyclic trend
- **D.** None of the above

36. Which is not an explanation for cyclic trend of disease?
- **A.** Environmental conditions
- **B.** Herd immunity variations
- **C.** Antigenic conditions
- **D.** Build up of susceptibles

37. All are true about propagated epidemic, *except:*
- **A.** No secondary peaks
- **B.** Due to person to person transmission
- **C.** Speed of spread depends upon herd immunity
- **D.** Depends upon attack rate

38. Objective of epidemic investigation is:
- **A.** To identify the cause and source of infection
- **B.** To determine factors responsible for occurrence of epidemic
- **C.** To define magnitude of epidemic outbreak
- **D.** All of the above

---

33 A 34 C 35 A 36 A 37 A 38 A

39. In investigation of an epidemic following steps be taken in consideration *except:*

A. Confirm the diagnosis

B. Isolation of cases

C. Study of ecological factors

D. Confirm that the epidemic exists

40. The area is declared free of epidemic:

A. No new case reported for six month since the last case

B. No new case reported for twice the incubation period of disease since the last case detected

C. Till the last secondary case recovers

D. No new case reported for the incubation period of the disease since the last case

41. When a disease frequency is measured over a period of several years of decades, it is called:

A. Secular trend

B. Seasonal trend

C. Cyclic trend

D. None of the above

---

39 B   40 B   41 A

Analytical Epidemiology

1. Analytical studies are undertaken to:
   A. Test the etiological hypothesis
   B. Screening the new cases in the community
   C. Identify high risk factors of the disease
   D. Determine the occurrence and distribution of disease

2. All the following are true regarding case control study *except:*
   A. It is suited for the evaluation of therapy or prophylaxis
   B. The study proceeds backwards from effect to cause
   C. The unit is the individual rather than the group
   D. Both exposure and outcome have occurred before the start of the study

3. Most important factor that should be considered while measuring exposure in case control study:
   A. Bias
   B. Matching
   C. Obtaining P-value
   D. Proper screening

4. Case control study is used for finding:
   A. Rare cause
   B. Incidence rate
   C. Multiple risk factors
   D. Morbidity rates

5. Causal association factor can be revealed by:
   A. Cohort study
   B. Case control study
   C. Cross sectional study
   D. Experimental study

---

1 A 2 A 3 A 4 C 5 B

6. **Case control study is used for study of:**
   - A. Common disease
   - B. Uncommon disease
   - C. Rare disease
   - D. Unknown disease

7. **Which of the following in case control studies ascertains whether there is statistical association between exposure status and occurrence of disease?**
   - A. Attributable risk
   - B. Odds ratio
   - C. P-value
   - D. Relative risk

8. **A case control study may have an advantage over a cohort study when the disease in question is:**
   - A. Fatal
   - B. Infections
   - C. Virulent
   - D. Rare

9. **All of the following are advantages of case control studies *except:***
   - A. Relative risk can be calculated
   - B. Useful in rare diseases
   - C. Odds ratio can be calculated
   - D. Cost effective and inexpensive

10. **Case control studies are useful for:**
    - A. Studying diseases that are rare
    - B. Estimating risk for an exposure
    - C. Generating casual hypothesis
    - D. All of the above

11. **All the following study designs are useful for hypothesis generation *except:***
    - A. Retrospective studies
    - B. Case control studies
    - C. Randomized controlled trials
    - D. Cross-sectional studies

---

6 C 7 C 8 D 9 A 10 D 11 B

12. Study of a person who has already contracted the disease:

A. Case control
B. Cohort
C. Control cohort
D. None or the above

13. All of the following features are true about case control study *except:*

A. No risk to subjects
B. Less prone to bias
C. Rapid and inexpensive
D. Risk factor can be identified -

14. In epidemiological studies important criterion for control group is that, it should be:

A. Equal in number
B. That the factor to be studied should be absent
C. Age and socioeconomic status matched
D. That the factor to be studied should be present

15. All are true about case control study *except:*

A. Provides information about natural history of disease
B. Uses comparison group to support an inference
C. Study proceeds backwards from effect to cause
D. Both exposure and disease have occurred before the start of study

16. Cross over study is done when:

A. Case and control are the same
B. Case and control are different
C. Control is same and case is different
D. Case is same and control is different

12 A **13 B** **14 B** **15 A** **16 A**

17. The most useful study in a hospital setting is:

A. Case control
B. Cohort
C. Cross-sectional
D. Longitudinal

18. Case control study is used for:

A. Finding multiple risk factors
B. Finding incidence rate
C. Finding a rare cause of disease
D. Finding prevalence rate

19. All are the advantages of case control study *except:*

A. Less chances of bias
B. Possible to study many diseases
C. Very economic
D. Less time consuming

17 A 18 A 19 A

fourteen

Assessment of Risk in Epidemiologic Studies

1. An independent risk factor is:

A. A factor that is associated with risk and is modifiable

B. A factor that is specific for the disease

C. A factor that can not be explained by and association with a second factor

D. A factor that is strongly related to chances of developing a disease

2. The importance of defining 'population at risk' in an epidemic is to:

A. Conduct survey

B. Prepare case sheet

C. Find death rate

D. Calculate attack rates

3. A risk factor is defined as:

A. A factor that causes the disease

B. A factor that places an individual at higher chance for developing the disease

C. A factor that is associated with risk and is modifiable

D. A factor that is specific for the disease

4. Which of the following is an odds ratio?

A. Relative risk

B. Proportional mortality rate

C. Association between risk factor and outcome

D. Ensure comparability between cases and controls

1 C 2 D 3 B 4 C

5. Odds ratio is derived from:
- **A.** Cross sectional study
- **B.** Case control study
- **C.** Randomized trial
- **D.** Cohort study

6. A cohort must have:
- **A.** Same year of birth
- **B.** Common place of residence
- **C.** Common disease history
- **D.** Passage through the same time period

7. In a Cohort study, the groups are compared on the basis of:
- **A.** Age
- **B.** Exposure status
- **C.** Inclusion or exclusion criteria
- **D.** Disease status

8. The natural history of disease is best established by:
- **A.** Retrospective study
- **B.** Prospective study
- **C.** Cross sectional study
- **D.** Cohort study

9. Which of the following is a measure of the risk of having a risk factor?
- **A.** Relative risk
- **B.** Risk ratio
- **C.** Odds ratio
- **D.** None of the above

10. Odds ratio is nearly the same as relative risk when:
- **A.** The risk factor is rare
- **B.** The disease is rare
- **C.** Odds ratio is calculated from a prospective study
- **D.** Relative risk is calculated from a retrospective study

---

5 B **6 D** **7 D** **8 D** **9 C** **10 B**

11. A double blind study of a vaccine is one in which:
- **A.** The study group receives the vaccine and the control group receives a placebo
- **B.** Neither observer nor subjects know the nature of placebo
- **C.** Neither the study group nor the control group knows the identity of the observer
- **D.** Neither observer nor subjects know which subject receives the vaccine and which receives a placebo

12. What is the main reason to use 'double blind' methods in a study?
- **A.** Minimize patients going off drug
- **B.** Reduce end point ascertainment bias
- **C.** Reduce observer measurement bias
- **D.** None of the above

13. The association between coronary artery disease (CAD) and smoking was found to be as follows:

CAD	**NO**	**CAD**
Smokers	**50**	**40**
Non smokers	**40**	**50**

The odds ratio can be estimated as:
- **A.** 1.56 **B.** 0.65
- **C.** 1.3 **D.** 1.75

14. Use of double blind trial is to:
- **A.** Avoid false negative results
- **B.** Avoid subject bias
- **C.** Avoid observer bias
- **D.** Increase true negatives

15. Which of the following is not true about cohort study:
- **A.** Study is short lived and technique is crude
- **B.** Prospective study
- **C.** Study proceeds from cause to effect
- **D.** Two groups should be comparable

---

11 D 12 C 13 A 14 B 15 A

16. All are true abort cohort study *except:*
   A. It is used when ample funds are available
   B. It is used when incidence of disease is very low among exposed
   C. It is used for the evidence of association between exposure and disease
   D. Groups should be equally susceptible

17. All are advantages of cohort study *except:*
   A. Bias is minimized
   B. Suitable for study of rare diseases
   C. Several possible outcomes related to exposure can be studied simultaneously
   D. Dose response ratio can be calculated

18. Bias is unlikely to invalidate cohort studies used to assess risk of exposure because:
   A. Exposure is usually determined prior to disease occurrence
   B. Actual relative risk can be determined
   C. Data collection is prospective
   D. In includes a large number of subjects

19. The likelihood of a causal relationship is increased by:
   A. Biological plausibility
   B. Temporal association
   C. Strength of association
   D. All of the above

20. Keeping the frequency of illness within acceptable limits is best described as disease:
   A. Surveillance
   B. Control
   C. Treatment
   D. Eradication

21. An odds ratio equals to one indicates that the association between the factors:
   A. Is low **B.** Is high
   C. Is perfect **D.** Does not exist

---

16 B 17 B 18 A 19 D 20 B 21 D

22. The role of control group in clinical trials is:
- **A.** To control the sampling error
- **B.** To control the size of the trial
- **C.** To control the placebo effect
- **D.** To control the uncertainties in the outcome

23. The strength of an association between a factor and a disease is best measured by:
- **A.** Attributable risk
- **B.** Relative risk
- **C.** Prevalence of the factor
- **D.** Incubation period

24. Odds ratio can be calculated from:
- **A.** Relative risk
- **B.** Attributable risk
- **C.** Incidence rate
- **D.** Prevalence rate

25. Which would be the best health statistic from the following in order to asses how strongly an exposure is related to a disease:
- **A.** Attributable risk
- **B.** Relative risk
- **C.** Incidence among the exposed
- **D.** Prevalence among the exposed

26. The ratio between the incidence among exposed and among non-exposed person is:
- **A.** Relative risk
- **B.** Causal risk
- **C.** Attributable risk
- **D.** Odds ratio

27. Relative risk can be obtained from:
- **A.** Case control study
- **B.** Retrospective study
- **C.** Prospective study
- **D.** Cross-sectional study

---

22 D 23 B 24 A 25 B 26 A 27 C

28. Relative risk is:

A. Risk among exposed ÷ risk in whole population

B. Risk among exposed ÷ risk in non exposed

C. Risk among exposed ÷ (risk among exposed – risk in non exposed)

D. Risk among exposed ÷ (risk among exposed + risk in non exposed)

29. Relative risk could show an association between:

A. Efficacy of two drugs

B. Altitude and endemic goitre

C. Oral contraception practice and pregnancy

D. Smoking and lung cancer

30. Relative risk of developing a disease is indicated by:

A. Incidence among exposed ÷ Incidence among non exposed

B. Incidence among exposed - Incidence among non exposed

C. Incidence among exposed ÷ Population at risk

D. None of the above

31. Relative risk could show an association between:

A. Smoking and lung cancer

B. OCP and pregnancy

C. Efficacy of two drugs

D. Altitude and endemic goiter

32. Relative risk is not the same as:

A. Risk ratio

B. Ratio of incidence rates

C. Risk difference

D. Risk in the exposed group related to the risk in unexposed group

---

28 B 29 B 30 A 31 A 32 C

33. Relative risk in a case control study is shown by which formula:

Risk factor	Developed disease	Did not develop disease
Present	a	b
Absent	c	d

A. $\frac{a}{ab} \div \frac{b}{cd}$ B. $\frac{a}{a+b} \div \frac{c}{c+d}$

C. $\frac{a}{a+c} \div \frac{b}{b+d}$ D. $\frac{a}{a+b} \div \frac{b}{c+d}$

34. Which of the following health statistics would be most useful in selecting risk factors to target for intervention in order to have the greatest health impact? When resources are limited:

A. Incidence of the disease among the exposed
B. Relative risk of the disease
C. Attributable risk
D. Prevalence of the disease among the exposed

35. Which one of the following measures is most useful in the generation of public health policy?

A. Attributable risk
B. Relative risk
C. Odds ratio
D. Population attributable risk percentage

36. Incidence of disease among exposed minus that of non-exposed is equal to:

A. Attributable risk
B. Relative risk
C. Odds ratio
D. None of the above

37. Attributable risk is not the same as:

A. Relative risk
B. Risk difference
C. Additional risk
D. Difference in incidence rates

---

33 B 34 C 35 D 36 A 37 A

38. Difference in incidence rate of disease between exposed group and non exposed group is:

A. Attributable risk
B. Relative risk
C. Risk ratio
D. Prevalence rate

39. The amount of disease that might be eliminated if the factor under study could be controlled can be indicated by:

A. Relative risk
B. Odds ratio
C. Attributable risk
D. Risk ratio

40. Which of the following is not true about odds ratio?

A. The odds ratio is always positive
B. The odd ratio is always more than one
C. The odds ratio can be three in some cases
D. The odds ratio can be 0.3 in some cases

38 A 39 C 40 B

Experimental Epidemiology

1. What is the 'gold standard' in medical research for evaluating the efficacy of new treatments?

A. Clinical trials
B. Case control study
C. Prospective study
D. Observational study

2. Which of the following is most cost effective method of establishing benefit of a treatment?

A. Case control study
B. Prospective clinical trial
C. Meta analysis
D. Retrospective study

3. The time interval between the primary and secondary case is:

A. Serial interval
B. Generation time
C. Median incubation period
D. Secondary attack rate

4. In an experiment to compare two treatments, subjects are allocated at random so that:

A. The sample may be referred to a known population
B. The experimenter will not know which treatment the subjects receive
C. The two groups will be as similar as possible apart from treatment
D. The subjects will get the treatment best suited to them

1 A 2 C 3 A 4 C

5. While analyzing a data, allocation into similar groups is done to ensure:

A. Accuracy
B. Sensitivity
C. Validity
D. Comparability

6. Temporal association between a risk factor and the disease relates to:

A. Cause and effect relationship
B. Duration and response relationship
C. Dose-response relationship
D. One to one relationship

7. In cause effect relationship the most essential criterion is:

A. Nature of relationship
B. Consistency of relationship
C. Strength of relationship
D. Duration of relationship

8. Longitudinal studies:

A. Are easy to conduct
B. Are very economic
C. Provide incidence of disease
D. Are good for studying single outcome

9. The 'placebo effect' observed in a study can be explained by:

A. Regression to the mean
B. Observer measurement bias
C. Unknown biologic effects to placebo
D. Increase study credibility

10. Which of the following factors is the most important to the validity of the conclusions drawn from a clinical trial?

A. Equal numbers of treated individuals an those given placebo
B. Effective randomization of participants
C. Followup of 100% of the participants
D. Inclusion in both groups of individuals of all ages

---

5 D   6 A   7 B   8 C   9 A   10 B

11. The number of patient required in a clinical trial to treat a specific disease increases as:
- **A.** The level of significance increases
- **B.** The drop out rate increases
- **C.** The incidence of the disease decreases
- **D.** The size of the expected treatment effect increases

12. Randomization is useful to eliminate:
- **A.** Observer bias
- **B.** Patient bias
- **C.** Confounding factors
- **D.** Sampling bias

13. Randomization and double blinding in a controlled trial are intended to accomplish of the following *except:*
- **A.** Minimize bias
- **B.** Reduce known confounding factors
- **C.** Optimize external validity
- **D.** Reduce unknown confounding factors

14. Which of the following statements describes the major advantages of a randomized clinical trial:
- **A.** It yields results replicable in other patients
- **B.** It rules out self selection of participants to the different treatment groups
- **C.** If enrolls representative patients
- **D.** It avoids observer bias

15. If there is no participation by 40% of study group, it is:
- **A.** Selection bias **B.** Response bias
- **C.** Subjective bias **D.** None of the above

16. A confounding variable in a statistical study is responsible for:
- **A.** Direct association
- **B.** Indirect association
- **C.** Temporal association
- **D.** Spurious association

11 B **12 C** **13 C** **14 A** **15 B** **16 B**

17. A confounding factor is defined as one:

A. Which is associated with exposure but not the disease

B. Which is associated with both disease and exposure

C. Which is associated with disease but not exposure

D. Which is not associated with both disease and exposure

18. Confounding bias in a case control study can be removed by:

A. Double blinding

B. Matching

C. By selecting representative population

D. By proper recalling events

19. Randomized controlled trial is a type of:

A. Experimental study
B. Case control study
C. Cohort study
D. Analytical study

20. All are true about randomized controlled trial *except:*

A. Avoidance of Intervention

B. Randomization

C. Selecting reference and experimental population

D. Experimental study

21. Randomization is:

A. Statistical procedure of allocating participants into study and control groups

B. Mixing different types of controls

C. Blinding is done to reduce bias

D. None of the above

22. Randomization into a clinical trial is best characterized by which of the following:

A. There is an equal chance of group assignment

B. Group assignment is unpredictable

C. Group assignment is unknown to the participant

D. Group assignment is sequential

---

17 B 18 B 19 A 20 A 21 A 22 B

23. What is the best method for ensuring that patients assigned to different study groups are similar in severity of disease at entry?

A. Randomization
B. Extensive baseline medical evaluations
C. Adjusting entry criteria
D. Blocking treatment assignments

24. The goal of randomized field trial is to determine vaccine effectiveness. Which of the following formula is correct for it?

A. Vaccine effectiveness (VE) = $\frac{\text{Attack rate}}{\text{(AR)}} \times 100$

B. $VE = \frac{\text{A R (Unvaccinated)} + \text{A R (Vaccinated)}}{\text{A R (Vaccinated)}} \times 100$

C. $VE = \frac{\text{A R (Unvaccinated)} + \text{A R (Vaccinated)}}{\text{A R (Unvaccinated)}} \times 100$

D. $VE = \frac{\text{A R (Vaccinated)} + \text{A R (Unvaccinated)}}{\text{Population at risk}} \times 100$

25. Which of the following interventions is appropriate to determine the efficacy of modified influenza vaccine for a particular year?

A. A randomized field trial
B. A retrospective cohort study
C. Routine surveillance
D. Review of data from previous years

26. When launching a study, many respondents are invited, some of them of whom fail to come; this is called:

A. Response bias
B. Selection bias
C. Volunteer bias
D. Berkesonian bias

23 A **24 C** **25 B** **26 C**

27. Randomization and Random Sampling are:
- **A.** Synonymous
- **B.** Different procedures
- **C.** Often amount to the same thing
- **D.** Substitutes to each other

28. The purpose of randomization in a clinical trial is:
- **A.** To bypass blinding
- **B.** To obviate the need of a placebo group
- **C.** To guard against ethical considerations
- **D.** To increase the likelihood of initial equivalence of groups

29. Matching can not be adopted in:
- **A.** Case control study
- **B.** Prospective study
- **C.** Randomized controlled trial
- **D.** Experiment

30. Which of the following is not true about non-randomized trial?
- **A.** High degree of comparability
- **B.** Approach is rather crude
- **C.** The experiment can utilize a natural control as itself
- **D.** Several trials may be needed before evaluation

31. Matching is done to avoid:
- **A.** Bias
- **B.** Observer variance
- **C.** Confounding factor
- **D.** Selection bias

32. The process of "matching" allows:
- **A.** Matching of factors in doubt
- **B.** Matched variables to be evaluated
- **C.** Selection of case and control with the same known confounding variables
- **D.** Avoid focusing on desired variables

33. Cross-matching is done in case control study to eliminate:
- **A.** Selection bias
- **B.** Relative risk
- **C.** Confounding factor
- **D.** Sampling error

27 B 28 D 29 C 30 A 31 C 32 A 33 C

Epidemiology

sixteen

Screening for Disease

1. In screening program, an effect comparable to the late look bias is called:

A. Recall bias
B. Selection bias
C. Spectrum bias
D. Length bias

2. Which one of the following characteristics of a diagnostic test is analogous to the statistical power of a study?

A. Positive predictive value
B. Negative predictive value
C. Sensitivity
D. Specificity

3. All of the following should be true of a disease for which screening is planned *except:*

A. The disease should be serious
B. The disease should be rare
C. the disease must be treatable
D. A population at risk should be identifiable

4. The usefulness of a screening test depends upon its:

A. Reliability
B. Sensitivity
C. Specificity
D. Predictivity

5. Screening is the most commonly used epidemiologicaľ tool in the school health services. Which level of prevention does it refer to?

A. Primary
B. Secondary
C. Tertiary
D. None of the above

1 D 2 C 3 B 4 B 5 A

6. **Amount of previously unrecognized disease that diagnosed as a result of screening effort is:**
   - A. Prevalence
   - B. Surveillance
   - C. Yield
   - D. Predictive value

7. **Selective screening refers to screening test applied to:**
   - A. Randomly selective group
   - B. Volunteers group
   - C. High risk group
   - D. None of the above

8. **Multi-phasic screening refers to:**
   - A. Application of two or more tests in combination
   - B. Applied to various places
   - C. Done at different time period and place
   - D. Test applied in various steps

9. **A good screening test must be:**
   - A. Acceptability
   - B. Repeatability
   - C. Validity
   - D. All of the above

10. **Repeatability of a screening test depends on:**
    - A. Biological variation
    - B. Observer variation
    - C. Instrumental error
    - D. All of the above

11. **Intra-observer variation can be minimized by:**
    - A. Taking the average of several replicate measurements at the same time
    - B. Intensive training of observers
    - C. Standardization of procedures for obtaining measurements
    - D. Repeated measurements overtime

12. **Validity of screening test is determined by:**
    - A. Accuracy
    - B. Predictive values of positive and negative tests
    - C. Sensitivity and specificity
    - D. Reliability

---

6 C 7 C 8 A 9 D 10 D 11 A
12 C

13. Specificity of test means, all *except:*
- **A.** Identifies those without disease
- **B.** True positive
- **C.** True negative
- **D.** An ideal screening test should have 100% specificity

14. Specificity is ability of a test to identify correctly:
- **A.** True negatives
- **B.** True positives
- **C.** False negatives
- **D.** False positive

15. Specificity of a test is:
- **A.** Ability to correctly identify those who have the disease
- **B.** Ability to correctly identify those who do not have the disease
- **C.** Identifies true positives
- **D.** Indicates the probability that a patient with positive result, actually has the disease

16. 95% specificity means:
- **A.** 95% of the diseased persons screened will give false negative result
- **B.** 5% of the non diseased persons screened by the test will give a true negative result
- **C.** 95% of the non diseased persons screened by the test will give a true negative result
- **D.** 5% of the diseased persons screened will give true positive result

17. All are factors influencing community diagnosis *except:*
- **A.** Age and sex distribution
- **B.** Incidence and Prevalence of disease
- **C.** Vital events
- **D.** Health measures taken

18. Specificity increases with:
- **A.** Increase in true positive
- **B.** Increase in true negative
- **C.** Increase in false negative
- **D.** Increase in false positive

13 B 14 A 15 B 16 C 17 D 18 B

19. The same screening test is applied to two communities A and B; B shows more false positive cases as compared to A. The possibility is:

A. B community has low prevalence
B. B community has high prevalence
C. High sensitivity
D. High specificity

20. Which is most economical and best screening:

A. Mass survey
B. Multiphasic screening
C. High risk screening
D. None of the above

21. The criteria for validity of a screening test is:

A. Sensitivity and specificity
B. Accuracy
C. Predictability
D. Cost effectiveness

22. Specificity increases with:

A. Increase in true positive
B. Increase in true negative
C. Increase in false positive
D. Increase in false negative

23. Predictive value of a positive test comprises all the following *except:*

A. Sensitivity **B.** Specificity
C. Disease incidence **D.** Disease prevalence

24. A cut off point:

A. Minimizes false positives
B. Minimizes false negatives
C. Maximizes true positives
D. Minimizes both false positives and false negatives

25. If the cut off point in the interpretation of the test is raised, one of the following may occur:

A. Sensitivity decreases and specificity increases
B. Sensitivity increases and specificity decreases
C. Sensitivity and specificity both increase
D. Sensitivity and specificity both decrease

19 A **20 C** **21 A** **22 B** **23 C** **24 D**
25 A

26. Positive predictive value of a test is:

Screening Test results	Diagnosis *Diseased*	*Not diseased*
Positive	a	b
Negative	c	d

A. $\frac{a\,d}{b\,c} \times 100$ B. $\frac{a}{a+b} \times 100$

C. $\frac{b}{a+b} \times 100$ D. $\frac{a+b}{c+d} \times 100$

27. Which of the following characteristics of a screening test is most effected by the prevalence of disease:

A. Sensitivity
B. Specificity
C. Predictive value
D. Likelihood ratio

28. Most important in screening test for community is:

A. Sensitivity
B. Specificity
C. Predictive value of positive test
D. Detectability

29. High prevalence of disease in ān area affects:

A. Sensitivity
B. Specificity
C. Predictive value
D. All of the above

30. Diagnostic power of a test to correctly exclude the disease is:

A. Sensitivity
B. Negative predictivity
C. Specificity
D. Positive predictivity

26 B 27 C 28 C 29 C 30 B

31. Predictive value of a positive test is:

A. $\frac{\text{True positive}}{\text{True positive + False positive}}$

B. $\frac{\text{True positive}}{\text{True positive + False negative}}$

C. $\frac{\text{False positive}}{\text{True positive + False negative}}$

D. $\frac{\text{True positive – False negative}}{\text{True positive + False positive}}$

32. Predictive value of a negative test is given by:

A. $\frac{\text{True negative}}{\text{True negative - False negative}}$

B. $\frac{\text{True negative}}{\text{True negative + False positive}}$

C. $\frac{\text{True negative}}{\text{True negative + False negative}}$

D. $\frac{\text{True negative – True positive}}{\text{True negative + False positive}}$

33. Percentage sensitivity of a test is:

A. $\frac{\text{True positive}}{\text{True positive + False positive}} \times 100$

B. $\frac{\text{True positive}}{\text{True positive + False negative}} \times 100$

C. $\frac{\text{True positive + True negative}}{\text{False positive + False negative}} \times 100$

D. $\frac{\text{False positive}}{\text{True negative + False positive}} \times 100$

31 A 32 C 33 B

34. Percentage specificity of a screening test is calculated by:

A. $\dfrac{\text{False positive}}{\text{True negative + False positive}} \times 00$

B. $\dfrac{\text{False negative}}{\text{True positive + False negative}} \times 100$

C. $\dfrac{\text{True negative}}{\text{True negative + False negative}} \times 100$

D. $\dfrac{\text{True negative}}{\text{True negative + False positive}} \times 100$

35. The sensitivity of a diagnostic test is its ability to detect:

A. Positive result in those who have disease
B. Positive result in those who do not have the disease
C. Negative result in those who have disease
D. Negative result in those who do not have the disease

36. Diagnostic power of the test is reflected by:

A. Sensitivity
B. Specificity
C. Predictive value
D. Population attributable risk

37. Predictive accuracy of a screening test depends on:

A. Sensitivity
B. Specificity
C. Disease prevalence
D. All of the above

38. An ideal screening test should have all *except:*

A. Low specificity **B.** High sensitivity
C. High specificity **D.** High yield

---

34 D 35 A 36 C 37 D 38 D

39. The best and the most economical method of screening for a disease is:

A. Mass screening
B. Prospective screening
C. High risk screening
D. Multiphasic screening

40. In a community identification of high risk individuals for coronary heart disease and the prevention of risk factor is:

A. Primary prevention
B. Surveillance
C. Multiphasic screening
D. Selective screening

41. More false positive cases in a community signify that the disease has:

A. High prevalence
B. High sensitivity
C. Low prevalence
D. Low sensitivity

---

39 C 40 D 41 C

Epidemiology

seventeen

Surveillance and Prevention of Disease

1. The most important function of sentinal surveillance is:

A. To determine the trend of disease in a population

B. To find the total amount of disease in a population

C. To plan effective control measures

D. To notify disease

2. Missing cases are detected by:

A. Active surveillance

B. Passive surveillance

C. Sentinal surveillance

D. Prevalence rate

3. Which of the following procedures is used for detection of missing contact:

A. Passive surveillance

B. Screening

C. Active surveillance

D. Continuous surveillance

4. Morbidity is measured by:

A. Active surveillance

B. Passive surveillance

C. Sentinal surveillance

D. Continuous surveillance

1 B 2 C 3 C 4 A

5. **Total morbidity is determined by:**
   A. Sentinal surveillance
   B. Active surveillance
   C. Passive surveillance
   D. Annual survey

6. **Primordial prevention is applied when:**
   A. Risk factors appear before disease
   B. No disease and no risk factors
   C. After risk factors appear
   D. Prevalence of disease is low

7. **Pap smear is an example of:**
   A. Primary level of prevention
   B. Secondary level of prevention
   C. Tertiary level of prevention
   D. None of the above

8. **Tertiary level of prevention is:**
   A. Rehabilitation
   B. Early diagnosis and treatment
   C. Health promotion
   D. Chemo prophylaxis

9. **Which type of prevention used in change of smoking habit:**
   A. Primordial B. Primary
   C. Secondary D. High risk strategy

10. **Serial interval is:**
    A. Gap between maximum and minimum incubation period
    B. Difference between sensitivity and specificity
    C. Time gap between primary and secondary cases
    D. Secondary attack rate

11. **Which one of the following is not a characteristic of non-communicable disease?**
    A. Multifactorial causation
    B. Long latent period
    C. Well defined etiological agent
    D. Variable onset

---

5 A 6 A 7 B 8 A 9 A 10 C
11 C

12. Prospective genetic counselling is the application of which level of prevention?

A. Primary
B. Secondary
C. Tertiary
D. Primordial

13. An example of secondary prevention is:

A. Vaccination against Hepatitis-B
B. Detection and treatment of hypertension
C. Early treatment of diabetic nephropathy
D. Harmone replacement therapy at menopause

14. The first case to come to the attention of the investigator is:

A. Primary case
B. Secondary case
C. Contact case
D. Index case

15. The first person becoming sick in an epidemic is called:

A. Index case
B. Contact case
C. Primary case
D. Secondary case

16. An agent with low pathogenicity and high infectivity would result in development of:

A. Carrier
B. Clinical case
C. Epidemic
D. Pandemic

17. Carriers are more dangerous than cases because they:

A. Increase duration of disease
B. Increase virulence
C. Infect more people
D. More infectious

18. Silent epidemic of the century is:

A. Coronary heart disease
B. Alzheimer's disease
C. Chronic liver disease
D. None of the above

---

12 A **13 B** **14 D** **15 C** **16 A** **17 C**
18 B

19. An out break is a:
A. Localized endemic
B. Localized epidemic
C. Localized pandemic
D. Localized exotic disease

20. The gap in time between the onset of the primary case and the secondary case is called:
A. Generation time
B. Latent period
C. Incubation period
D. Serial interval

21. The period between the entry of organism in the host and appearance of signs and symptoms is called:
A. Period of surveillance
B. Incubation period
C. Latent period
D. None of the above

22. Incubation period is useful to determine:
A. The source of infection
B. The prognosis of disease
C. The period of surveillance
D. All of the above

23. Incubation period is helpful for all *except:*
A. Isolation
B. Source identification
C. Quarantine
D. Preventive immunization

24. In control of communication diseases, the period of quarantine in respect of a disease is determined by:
A. Duration of illness
B. Incubation period
C. Carrier state
D. Infectivity period

---

19 B 20 D 21 B 22 D 23 A 24 B

25. In control of communicable disease the period of quarantine in respect of a disease is determined by:

A. Incubation period B. Duration of disease
C. Carrier state D. Infectivity period

26. All are true about common source epidemic *except:*

A. Children are more affected
B. Abrupt end
C. Acute onset
D. Large number of cases in same time

27. Prophylactic administration of vitamin A in a child is:

A. Specific protection
B. Rehabilitation
C. Early treatment
D. Health promotion

28. First step in investigation of epidemic:

A. Confirm diagnosis B. Find the source
C. Sanitation D. Spot map

29. The first step for conducting an epidemic investigation is to:

A. Determine the case count
B. Calculate the incubation period
C. Verify the diagnosis
D. Determine the population at risk

30. Sullivan's Index measures:

A. Morbidity B. Mortality
C. Disability D. Infectivity

31. Health surveillance is:

A. A systemic collection of health data
B. Active reporting of diseases
C. Continuous scrutiny of all aspects of occurrence and spread of disease
D. Investigation and follow up

---

25 A 26 A 27 A 28 A 29 C 30 C
31 C

32. Most important epidemiological tool used for assessing disability in children is:

A. ADL (activities of daily living)
B. PQLI
C. DALY's
D. IQ tests

33. All are true about active immunity *except:*

A. Immunity is rapidly established
B. Severe reactions are rare
C. Duration of protection is long lasting
D. Protective efficacy is more

34. Herd immunity depends on:

A. Herd structure
B. Immunization status of herd
C. Sub-clinical infection
D. All of the above

35. Active and passive immunity is given simultaneously for the following *except:*

A. Tetanus
B. Measles
C. Rabies
D. Hepatitis-B

36. Host in which parasite attains maturity or passes in sexual stage is called:

A. Secondary host
B. Intermediate host
C. Definitive host
D. Facultative host

37. Hospital acquired infection is:

A. Nosocomial
B. Contagious
C. Water borne
D. Opportunistic

38. Natural habitat in which the organism metabolizes and replicates is:

A. Reservoir
B. Carrier
C. Vector
D. Source of infection

---

32 A 33 A 34 D 35 B 36 C 37 A
38 A

39. All are true about sub-clinic cases *except:*
   A. Host does not shed the infectious agent
   B. Can be detected only by laboratory tests
   C. Play a dominant role in maintaining endemicity in the community
   D. Responsible for immunity shown by person to a variety of disease producing organisms

40. Indirect transmission occurs by all *except:*
   A. Air **B.** Water
   C. Transplacental **D.** Vector

41. Most common mode of transmission of nosocomial infection is:
   A. Formite borne **B.** Air borne
   C. Vector borne **D.** Vehicle borne

42. Antecedent factor can not be:
   A. Death **B.** Exposure
   C. Infection **D.** Risk factor

43. True about vehicle transmission is:
   A. Common source of infection after traceable
   B. Higher the dose, higher the number of cases
   C. Not always possible to isolate organism from vehicle
   D. All the above

44. Emporiatrics refers to:
   A. Health of travelers
   B. Occupational hazards
   C. Air pollution
   D. Environment

45. Which of the following is true about exotic disease?
   A. Outbreak of disease in given population
   B. Disease transmitted to men from animals
   C. Disease newly imported into a country
   D. Disease transmitted from man to man

---

39 A 40 C 41 B 42 A 43 D 44 A
45 C

46. Quarantine is for:
A. Generation time
B. Shortest incubation period
C. Longest incubation period
D. Infective period

47. The best method of promoting healthy life in children is:
A. Primordial prevention
B. Propagated epidemic
C. Modern epidemic
D. Continuous epidemic

48. Prevention of emergence of risk factor is:
A. Primary prevention
B. Primordial prevention
C. Secondary prevention
D. Tertiary prevention

49. Primary prevention does not include:
A. Early diagnosis and treatment
B. Specific protection
C. Health promotion
D. Health education

50. Virulence of disease is indicated by:
A. Proportional mortality rate
B. Specific mortality rate
C. Case fatality ratio
D. Amount of GDP spent on the disease

51. Primordial prevention is done in population:
A. Without risk factors
B. With risk factors
C. With low prevalence of disease
D. With disease

52. Killed bacterial vaccine is:
A. Pertussis
B. BCG
C. Diphtheria
D. Toxoid

46 C 47 A 48 B 49 A 50 C 51 A
52 A

53. The following diseases are under surveillance of WHO, *except:*
- A. Tuberculosis
- B. Plague
- C. Malaria
- D. Relapsing fever

54. Notifiable disease is:
- A. Cholera
- B. Influenza
- C. Malaria
- D. Varicella

55. All are live vaccines, *except:*
- A. Pertussis
- B. Measles
- C. BCG
- D. Typhoid oral

56. Vector control means:
- A. Control of cattle and pets
- B. Control of mosquito breeding places
- C. Destruction of street dogs
- D. All of the above

57. Which of the following statements is true about sporadic?
- A. Unusual occurrence of disease in excess of expected occurrence
- B. Haphazard occurrence of disease from time to time
- C. Constant presence of disease in given population
- D. None of the above

58. Itch mite is an example of:
- A. Infestation
- B. Infection
- C. Contamination
- D. Colonization

---

53 A 54 A 55 A 56 D 57 B 58 A

59. Cold chain refers to:

A. Very cold temperature
B. Epidemic of influenza
C. Cold and flu-fever
D. Storage and transport of vaccine at low temperature

60. Most heat sensitive vaccine is:

A. Polio
B. Measles
C. BCG
D. TT

61. Surveillance is necessary for all recommended by WHO, *except:*

A. TB
B. Malaria
C. Plague
D. Relapsing Fever

62. True about Ring vaccination:

A. Given around 100 yards of a case detected
B. Given to produce a ring shaped lesion
C. Given around a mile of a case detected
D. Given by a ring shaped machine

---

59 D 60 A 61 A 62 A